Meriam Khadhar
Sahara Bouassida
Rim Goucha

Berger's disease:

Meriam Khadhar
Sahara Bouassida
Rim Goucha

Berger's disease:

overview

ScienciaScripts

Imprint

Cover image: www.ingimage.com

This book is a translation from the original published under ISBN 978-620-6-72432-2.

Publisher:
Sciencia Scripts
is a trademark of
Dodo Books Indian Ocean Ltd. and OmniScriptum S.R.L publishing group

120 High Road, East Finchley, London, N2 9ED, United Kingdom
Str. Armeneasca 28/1, office 1, Chisinau MD-2012, Republic of Moldova, Europe
Printed at: see last page
ISBN: 978-620-8-24579-5

Contents

Chapter 1

Immunoglobulin A nephropathy is a chronic glomerulonephritis characterised by the presence of predominant and diffuse immunoglobulin A (IgA) deposits on direct immunofluorescence (DIF) renal biopsy (RBB)(1).

Elie encompasses Berger's disease, IgA vasculitis (rheumatoid purpura) and IgA secondary nephropathies (Appendix 1).

Primary IgA nephropathy (NIgA) was first described in 1968 by Berger and Hinglais (2).

It is the most common primitive glomerulonephritis in the world (3).

Much progress has been made in understanding the pathophysiological mechanisms of NIgA, suggesting an abnormality in IgA synthesis or metabolism secondary to an autoimmune mechanism influenced by genetic and environmental factors(4).

Primary IgA nephropathy can occur at any age. The male/female sex ratio varies between nations (1). The clinical and biological manifestations vary, from completely asymptomatic forms revealed by routine urinary examinations (school or employment visits) to severe forms revealed by rapidly progressive renal failure. Classically, however, NIgA is revealed by macroscopic haematuria concomitant with upper respiratory tract infections. Arterial hypertension is common and is frequently associated with hematuria in this type of nephropathy.

Several histological classifications have been proposed, the most recent of which is the Oxford classification (5,6).

Treatment of NIgA is essentially based on nephroprotective therapy (7).

Primary NIgA is characterised by a variable course, with the possibility of complete clinical remission or progression to end-stage renal disease (ESRD) in 30 to 40% of cases (8).

The great difficulty in this disease lies in predicting and identifying renal prognostic factors.

This prompted us to carry out a retrospective study with the following objectives:

- To estimate the incidence of primary IgA nephropathy in the series of the internal medicine A department at the Charles Nicolle hospital in Tunis during the period from 1992 to 2021.
- Specify its epidemiological, clinico-biological, histological and therapeutic features.
- Study renal survival as a function of clinical, biological, histological and therapeutic data.

Chapter 2

1. PATIENTS :

1.1. Type of study :

We conducted a retrospective descriptive, analytical and comparative study based on the records of patients hospitalised in the internal medicine A department of the Charles Nicolle Hospital in Tunis over a period of 30 consecutive years between 1992 and 2021 and presenting with primary IgA nephropathy (NIgA) (Berger's disease).

1.2. Inclusion criteria :

In this study, we included patients aged over 15 years with IgA nephropathy confirmed by renal biopsy and considered to be primary in the presence of a negative etiological work-up.

1.3. Non-inclusion criteria :

- Patients with secondary NIgA (Appendix 1)
- Patients with IgA vasculitis (rheumatoid purpura)

1.4. Exclusion criteria

They were excluded from the study:

- Patients whose records were unusable or lost.

The patient selection stages are shown in this flow chart.

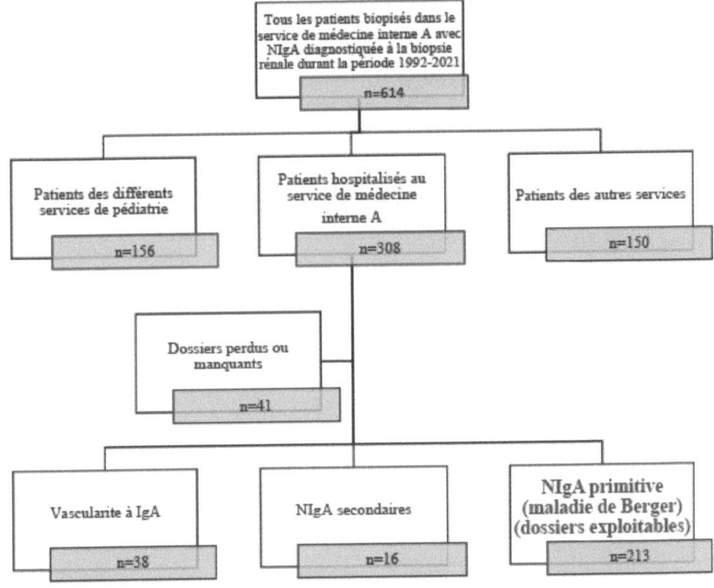

Figure 1: Flow diagram of the population studied

2. Methods :

2.1. Data collection :

We selected patients with IgA nephropathy confirmed on renal biopsy with positive immunofluorescence (IF) and negative etiological investigation.

We first drew up an information sheet which enabled us to record the following data from the patients' medical records and biopsy results (Appendix 2):

2.1.1. Epidemiological data:

For each case, we collected epidemiological data on age, gender, geographical origin, level of education and professional status.

2.1.2. Anamnesis data:

We specified the presence or absence of familial consanguinity, and the presence of a family history of nephropathy, hematuria or arterial hypertension (AH).

We looked for the presence of personal antecedents of hematuria and its type (microscopic or macroscopic), the notion of repeated ENT infections, the presence of diabetes and antecedents of cardiopathy, hypertension and allergy. We noted the patient's smoking habits and number of pack-years (PA), alcohol consumption and drug addiction.

We have specified the triggering factors and the time interval between these factors and the first signs of the disease.

2.1.3. Clinical data:

We looked for these elements:

- Weight (Kg), height (cm)
- The patient's BMI (kg/m):^{2}

The body mass index (BMI) was calculated using the following formula:

- BMI (kg/m2) = weight/height^{2}

The World Health Organisation (WHO) classification of BMI is shown in Table I (9).

Table I: Classification of Г1MC according to the World Health Organization

BMI (kg/m2)	*Interpretation*
<18.5 Between 18.5 and 25 Between 25 and 30 >30	Underweight Normal build Overweight Obese

BMI: Body Mass Index

- Urine test strip results:

Microscopic haematuria is defined as haematuria measured with a urine dipstick in terms of the number of crosses.

Macroscopic haematuria is defined as the emission of frankly haematic urine at 1'mil nu, corresponding to a red cell count >300,000 cells/ml.

- Measuring blood pressure :

Hypertension is defined as a systolic blood pressure (SBP) value >140 mmHg and/or a diastolic blood pressure (DBP) value >90 mmHg(10).

Table II: Grade of hypertension

Categories	*PAS (mmHg)*	*DBP (mmHg)*	
Grade 1	140-159	And/or	90-99
Grade 2	160-179	And/or	100-109
Grade 3	>180	And/or	>110
Systolic hypertension	>140	And	<90

SAP: systolic blood pressure; DBP: diastolic blood pressure

- The presence or absence of extra-renal signs (skin, respiratory, joint, digestive)

2.1.4. Biological data:

2.1.4.1. Laproteinuria:

Pathological proteinuria is defined as a value greater than or equal to 0.3g/24h.

2.1.4.2. Nephrotic syndrome:

The nephrotic syndrome has a purely biological definition. It is defined by the following triad:(11)

- Proteinuria greater than or equal to 3g/24 hours.
- Protein levels below 60g/l.
- An albuminemia of less than 30g/l.

It is compromised by the presence of arterial hypertension and/or haematuria and/or organic renal failure.

2.1.4.3. Renal function:

Renal function is assessed by measuring creatinineemia and glomerular filtration rate (GFR), which is calculated using the Modification of Diet in Renal Disease (MDRD) equation(12,13).

eDFG = 175 x (S_{cr} x 0.01 I3) '-^{154} x ige °"^{201} x 0.742 (if female) x 1.212 (if black)

Chronic renal failure (CRF) is defined as a GFR of less than 60ml/min/l,73 m^2 body surface area (BSA) for at least 3 months.

The stages of chronic kidney disease (CKD) have been defined according to the KDIGO 2012 (Kidney Disease Improving Global Outcomes) recommendations(14)(Table III).

Table III: Stages of chronic kidney disease

GFR stage (ml/mn/1.73 m2)		*Definition*
1	>90	Chronic kidney disease* with normal or increased GFR**.
2	60-89	Chronic kidney disease* with slightly reduced GFR
3A	45- 59	Chronic renal failure
3B	30- 44	moderee
4	15-29	Severe chronic renal failure
5	<15	Chronic end-stage renal failure

*With markers of renal damage: proteinuria, Иёта1иг1е, leukocyturia and/or morphological and/or histological abnormalities and/or markers of tubular dysfunction, persisting for more than 3 months.
**DFG: C^bit of filtration д1отёги1аке.

2.1.4.4. Blood count (CBC) :

Anemia is defined as a hemoglobin level of <13 g/dl in men and <12 g/dl in women.
Thrombocytopenia is defined as a platelet count < 150,000/mm .^{3}

Hyperleukocytosis is defined as a white blood cell count >10000/mm .[3]

2.1.4.5. *Cytobacteriological examination of urine (ECBU)*

Leukocyturia is defined biologically as a leukocyte count >10,000/ml.

Haematuria is defined as red blood cells greater than 0,000/ml on ECBU.

Bacteriuria is defined as germs in excess of 100,000/ml.

2.1.4.6. *Lipid profile:*

Hypercholesterolemia is defined, according to laboratory standards, as a plasma cholesterol level above 5.5 mmol/1.

Hypertriglyceridemia is defined by laboratory standards as a blood triglyceride level above al.7 mmol/1.

2.1.4.7. *Uricemia:*

Hyperuricemia is defined as a uric acid level > 420 mmol/1 in men and > 360 mmol/1 in women.

2.1.5. Imaging and specialist examinations:

- Renal ultrasound: we noted the size of both kidneys and the corticomedullary differentiation.
- Cardiac ultrasound: we assessed the left ventricular ejection fraction (LVEF) and the presence or absence of pericardial effusion.
- Chest X-ray: we looked for pneumopathy, cardiomegaly or pleural effusion.

2.1.6. Anatomopathological study:

The renal biopsy was performed in the pathology laboratory of Internal Medicine A and in the radiology department. The time taken to perform the biopsy was specified in relation to the onset of symptoms. In the absence of contraindications, the sample was taken under ultrasound or CT scan percutaneously. Puncture was performed under local anaesthetic using a 14 G Vim-Silverman needle until 2014, when the 14 or 16 G single-use gun was introduced. Two fragments were taken, one for light microscopy (OM) and the second for IFD.

- Study in MO :

The collected fragment was fixed in Dubose Brasil liquid for 4 hours and then dehydrated in alcohol baths of increasing concentration (70°, 90° and absolute alcohol). It was then placed in a toluene bath and then in liquid paraffin at 60°C for 2 hours and 30 minutes. Finally, the oriented biopsy was embedded in a mould.

Sections were cut using the Leitz 1512 microtome to a thickness of 2pm (4pm for sections intended for Congo red staining). Elies were mounted on slides.

Five stains were used for each PBR:

- Masson trichrome staining.
- Staining with hematein and eosin.
- Wilder's reticulin staining modified by Callard.
- Staining with Schiff's periodic acid (PAS).
- Systematic colouring in the Rouge Congo.
- IFD study :

Fragments for immunofluorescence were frozen at minus 20°C and then cut using a cryostat. They were subjected to a direct immunofluorescence technique in the presence of the following antisera: anti IgG, anti IgA, anti IgM, anti C3, anti Clq, anti fibrinogenes, anti Kappa light chains and anti Lambda light chains.

- Electron microscopy (EM) study

As part of a research protocol, we carried out an ME study on certain patients. Fragments intended for ME were immersed in glutaradehyde fixative and then in sodium cacodylate buffer. This was followed by post-fixation in 2% osmic acid. The fragments were dehydrated in ethanol baths and then impregnated with epoxy resin. The biopsies were cut to a thickness of 1 pm in order to select the areas of interest on which ultra-thin 70-80 nm sections would be taken.

Two stains were used: uranyl acetate and lead citrate.

- Analysis:

The diagnosis of NIgA was based on the presence of predominantly mesangial lgA deposits on IFD.

We used the data provided by the PBR report to describe the glomerular, tubular and vascular lesions, as well as the deposits observed on IFD. In our early biopsy reports, the term 'fibrous endarteritis' was used to describe vascular lesions of small-calibre arteries. Currently, in the literature, the term "arteriosclerosis" is used to describe these lesions. In order to harmonise our work, we have adopted the term "arteriosclerosis" throughout the series.

Prior to 2009, we used the HAAS classification to classify biopsies. Subsequently, we reclassified all biopsies according to the MEST-C score.

- **Oxford classification:(15)**

The Oxford classification is NIgA's second histological classification. It was proposed in 2009 by an international working group of nephrologists and pathologists from ten different countries (5). They selected the following anatomopathological lesions: mesangial proliferation (M), segmental glomerulosclerosis (S), endocapillary hypercellularity (E) and extent of interstitial fibrosis/tubular atrophy (T). This classification has been validated in the European population (16) and in the North American population (17). In 2017, they added another criterion to this classification, which is the presence or absence of crescents (C)(18) (Table IV).

Table IV: Oxford classification and MEST-C score

Variable Histopathological	*Definition*	*Score*
Mesangial proliferation (M)	Presence of more than four cells in a mesangial axis.	MO: in 50% or less of glomeruli. Ml: in more than 50% of glomeruli.
Endocapillary proliferation(E)	Presence of cells in the lumen of glomerular capillaries reducing this lumen	E0: absent El : present
Segmental glomerulosclerosis (S)	Sclerosis of part of the flocculus or flocculocapsular synechiae	SO: absent IF: present
Tubular	Percentage of affected cortical	TO: 0-25% of the cortical

atrophy/interstitial fibrosis (T)	surface with tubular atrophy or interstitial fibrosis	surface T1: 26-50% of cortical surface area T2: > 50% of the cortical surface
Cellular / fibro-cellular crescents (C)	Extra-capillary proliferation Cellular or fibro-cellular growth	CO: No crescents Cl: Crescents in less than 25% of glomeruli C2: Crescents in 25% or more of glomeruli

- Post-PBR complications:

We have reported on all complications arising after renal biopsy.

2.1.7. Treatment:

We have precise information for each patient:

- Non-medicinal treatments include tonsillectomy, fish oil, a low-salt diet, a lipid-lowering diet and smoking cessation.
- Drug treatments received:
- **Antihypertensives and their classes**
- **Corticoids** (the protocol used is oral corticotherapy or the Pozzi protocol)

Pozzi's protocol consists of (19):

- Three doses of 1 g of methylprednisolone over three consecutive days at the first, 3[eme] and 5[eme] months.
- Followed by oral prednisone (0.5 mg/kg every other day) for six months.

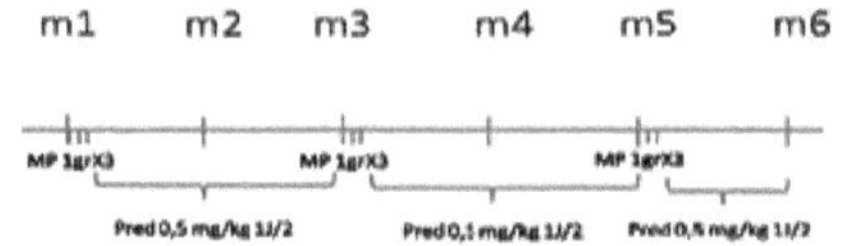

M: Month; D:day; MP: methylprednisolone; pred: oral prednisone.

Figure 2: Pozzi protocol

Indications of the Pozzi protocol :

> Persistent proteinuria greater than lg/24h after three months of nephroprotective treatment.

> Creatinemia <133pmol/l.

Use of the Pozzi protocol began in 2007 in our department.

> **Other immunosuppressants** (Doses and indications for prescription)

2.1.8. Evolution:

For each patient, we collected the following evolutionary elements:

- Duration of follow-up and compliance with treatment.
- Clinical-biological parameters: systolic blood pressure (SBP) and diastolic blood pressure (DBP), haematuria, 24-hour proteinuria, urine and creatinemia at 1 month, 3 months, 6 months, 1 year, 18 months, 2 years and at the end of follow-up.

- Whether or not the disease has reached the terminal stage and the time taken to reach it.
- The need for extra-renal purification: type, time to dialysis.
- Renal transplantation (RT): type of donor, HLA of donor and recipient with number of mismatches, time from RT to end stage, induction and maintenance treatment, outcome, need for graft biopsy and outcome.
- Death and its cause.

2.2. Statistical study :

The data collected were analysed using version 24 of SPSS for Windows (Statistical Package for Social Science: SPSS Inc, Chicago, IL).

2.2.1. Descriptive study:

The analysis was based on the calculation of simple frequencies and relative frequencies (percentages) for the qualitative variables, and on the calculation of means, medians, standard deviations and range (extreme values = minimum and maximum) for the quantitative variables. The results were presented in the form of summary tables, histograms and pie charts.

2.2.2. Analytical and comparative study:

Qualitative variables were compared using Pearson's chi-square test and, if necessary, Fisher's two-tailed exact test, depending on the conditions under which these tests were applied. Quantitative variables were compared using the Student's t-test or the MacNemar test, depending on the distribution of the variable.

Survival data were studied by establishing a survival curve using the Kaplan Meier method.

The search for prognostic factors for survival was carried out in a univariate analysis (factor by factor) by comparing the survival curves using the Log rank test.

The multivariate analysis was based on binary logistic regression adjusted for variables significantly associated with the event under study and identified by univariate analysis, as well as variables described in the literature.

In all statistical tests, the significance level was set at 0.05.

We also carried out a comparative analysis between the two periods of our study: the first period from 1992-2006 and the second period from 20072021.

2.3. Bibliographic research :

We based our work on the results of published articles, theses and abstracts. To do this, we used several sites: Science direct, PubMed and the Google scholar search engine.

The keywords used were: IgA nephropathy, Berger's disease, epidemiology, evolution, Oxford classification.

Bibliographic references were managed using the "Mendeley reference manager" software.

2.4. Conflict of interest:

We have no conflict of interest.

3. DEFINITIONS :

3.1. IgA vasculitis :

IgA vasculitis, known as rheumatoid purpura, is a systemic vasculitis of the small vessels with deposits of immunoglobulin A (IgA) (1). It is characterised by the association of cutaneous vascular purpura with joint and gastrointestinal signs. Renal involvement is sometimes associated with these signs. This is glomerulonephritis with lgA mesangial deposits (1).

3.2. Secondary IgA nephropathy :

Several secondary causes of IgA nephropathy have been reported in the literature (20): hepatic, inflammatory, autoimmune, lymphoproliferative, neoplastic and infectious diseases, in particular HIV (Appendix 1).

3.3. Recurrence on the graft :

Recurrence of NIgA is characterised by the reappearance of proteinuria and microscopic haematuria in the majority of cases, in transplant patients with diffuse lgA deposits and/or histological lesions (21). Elie may be a cause of graft loss in 5-10% of cases.

Chapter 3

1. DESCRIPTIVE STUDY :

1.1. Epidemiological characteristics :

1.1.1. Incidence:

During the period from 1992 to 2021, and after eliminating lost records and records of patients not hospitalised in Internal Medicine Department A, we selected 213 adult patients with primary IgA nephropathy for our study.

The average incidence of IgA nephropathy was 7 new cases per year. The incidence of IgA nephropathy during the study period is shown in Figure 3.

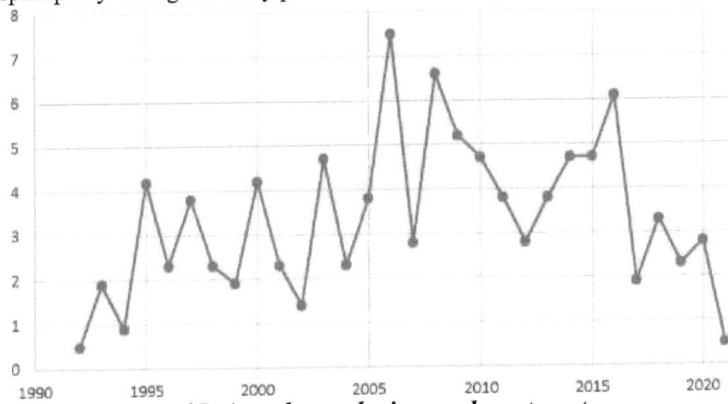

Figure 3: Incidence of IgA nephropathy in our department

1.1.2. Age at diagnosis :

The mean age of patients at diagnosis was 34 ± 12 years, with extremes ranging from 15 to 80 years. The age range was predominantly between 21 and 30 years. The age distribution was as follows:

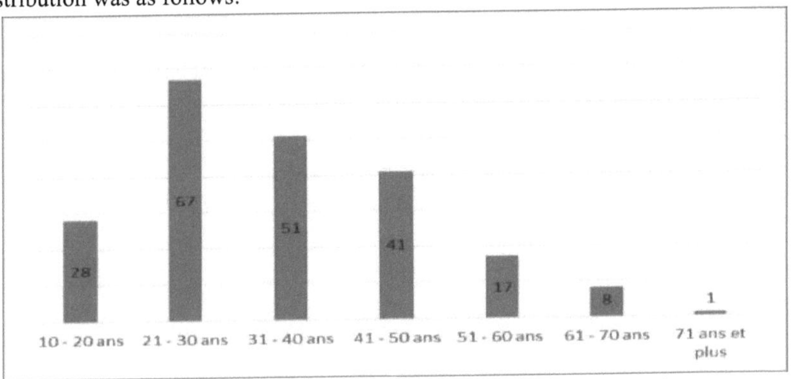

Figure 4 : Breakdown of patients by age at diagnosis

1.1.3. Legenre:

We noted a predominance of men (136 men/77 women) with a sex ratio of al.77.

1.1.4. Geographical origin:

All the patients were North African. They were mainly from the north of the country (85%), more specifically from the capital (34.7%). The other patients were from the centre (6.5%) and the south (8%). Only one patient was from Libya.

1.1.5. Level of education and professional status:

Twenty-six patients had university level education (12.2%), eighty-nine patients had secondary level education (41.8%), thirteen of whom had reached baccalaureate level (6.1%), eighty-one had primary level education (38%) and seventeen were illiterate (8%).

The breakdown by professional status was as follows: (Table V)

Table V: Breakdown of patients by professional status

Professional status	*Frequency*	*Percentage (%)*
In training	26	12,2
Assets	132	62
No profession	49	23
Retirement	6	2,8
Total	213	100

2. CLINICAL STUDY :

2.1. Family history :

- Arterial hypertension :

High blood pressure was reported in the siblings, ascendants or descendants of 96 patients (45.1%).

- Diabetes :

We found a family history of diabetes in 31 patients (14%).

- Nephropathy :

Macroscopic haematuria in family members was noted in 12 patients (5%).

Familial nephropathy was diagnosed in 39 cases. Among the familial cases, fifteen were in the renal replacement stage (RRT) and three had undergone renal transplantation.

We diagnosed familial IgA nephropathy in four patients. The discovery of this nephropathy was part of a work-up for organ donation in three cases, and as part of an investigation into advanced renal failure in another.

- Neoplasia :

Six patients reported a family history of neoplasia.

2.2. Parental consanguinity :

We found parental consanguinity in 61 patients (28%). The degree of consanguinity was not specified in the majority of cases.

2.3. Personal history:

- Forty-two patients (19.7%) had a history of recurrent ENT infections.
- The notion of one or more episodes of unexplained macroscopic haematuria was found in 56 patients (26%).

- Allergy was reported by 15 patients (7%).
- With regard to gynaeco-obstetric antecedents, three patients had a history of recurrent aborted pregnancies and one patient had reported fetal death in utero. All patients had negative anti-cardiolipin antibodies, anti-beta-2-glycoproteins and circulating anti-coagulants.

Other personal antecedents are summarised in Figure 5.

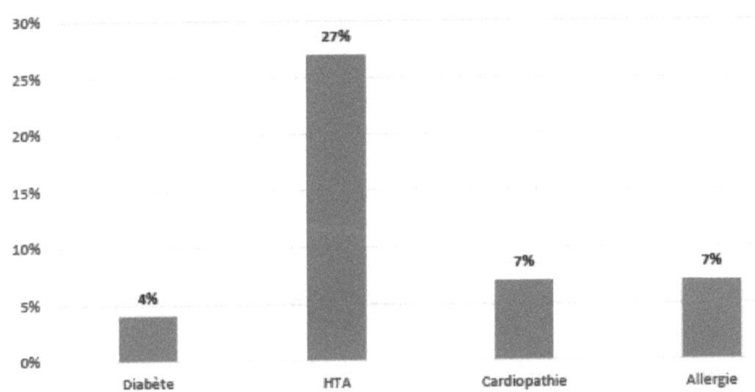

Figure 5: Personal antecedents of our population

2.4. Lifestyle habits :

Eighty-seven patients were smokers (40.8%), with an average of 16 smokes.
Alcohol consumption was reported in five patients.
Drug addiction was noted in two patients. The type of addiction was not specified.

2.5. Circumstances of discovery :

The most frequent reason for discovery was hypertension (25.4%). The circumstances of discovery are shown in Table VI.

Table VI: Distribution of the population studied according to the circumstances of discovery of IgA nephropathy

Circumstances of discovery	*Frequency*	*Percentage (%)*
ffidemes	25	11,7
Arterial hypertension	**54**	**25,4**
Macroscopic hematuria	40	18,8
Incidental: urine sediment anomalies	26	12,2
Nephrotic syndrome	31	14,5
Renal insufficiency	37	17,4

2.6. Triggering factors:

The presence of triggers for IgA nephropathy was noted in 65 cases (30.5%) (table VII).

Table VII: Breakdown of patients by triggering factor

Triggering factors	*Frequency*	*Percentage (%)*

Infection	56	26,3
Taking medication	1	0,5
Pregnancy	8	3,7
Not found	148	69,5
Total	213	100

An episode of ENT infection preceding the onset of the disease was found in 73% of cases. The distribution of patients by type of infection was as follows (Figure 6):

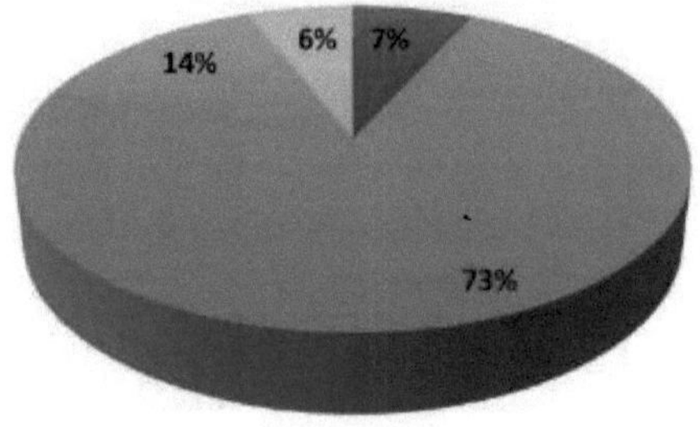

Figure 6: Breakdown of patients by type of infection

The median time between infection and first symptomatology was 0.5 days, with extremes of 0 and 60 days.

2.7. Clinical examination at the time of hospitalisation :

2.7.1. General signs:

Nine patients (4.2%) had an alteration in general condition. Fever was observed in 6 patients (2.8%).

2.7.2 Body mass index (BMI) :

The mean weight was 71.5 ± 15.2 kg, with extremes ranging from 42 to 8 kg.

The mean height was 167.9 ± 8.8 cm, with extremes ranging from 145 to 90 cm.

The median BMI was 24.6 kg/m^2 with extremes between 16.7 and 42.58 kg/m^2 . The distribution according to BMI was as follows (Figure 7).

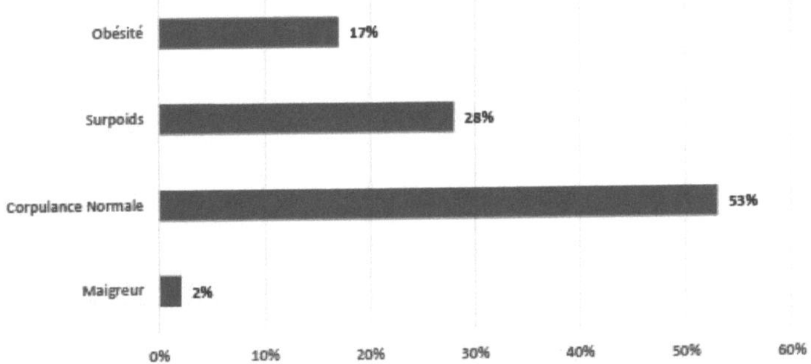

Figure 7: Distribution of patients by body mass index

1.1.3. Arterial pressure:

The median systolic blood pressure was 150 mmHg, with extremes between 90 and 250 mmHg.

The median diastolic blood pressure was 90 mmHg, with extremes between 50 and 140 mmHg.

Hypertension was present in 109 patients (51%) at the time of hospitalisation. Severe grade 3 hypertension was present in 39% of cases (Figure 8).

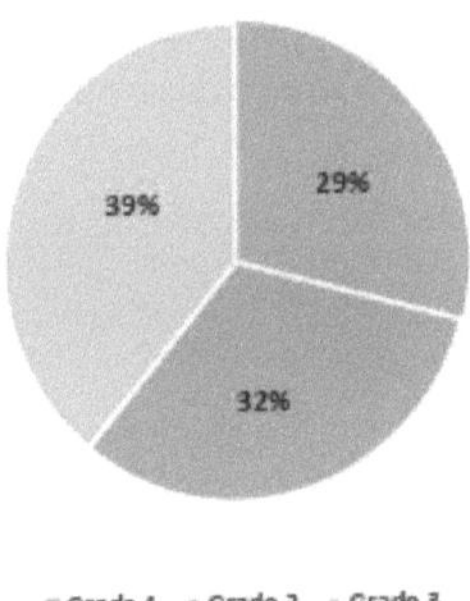

Figure 8: Grade of initial hypertension in our population

1.1.4. Kidney signs:

Eighty-five patients (39.9%) had renal-type redemas of the lower limbs; bilateral soft whites retaining the bucket and declining.

On admission, macroscopic and microscopic haematuria were observed in 36 patients (17%) and 137 patients (64.3%).

Forty patients (18.7%) had no hematuria.

Significant proteinuria at three crosses was observed in 49.8% of patients.

The results of the dipstick test are summarised in Table VIII.

Table VIII: Distribution of patients according to the number of crosses for hematuria and proteinuria on dipstick examination

	Cross	Frequency	Percentage (%)
Hematuria	0	40	18,8
	1	28	13,1
	2	39	18,3
	3	**106**	**49,8**
Proteinuria	0	7	3,3
	1	38	17,8
	2	62	29,1
	3	**106**	**49,8**

1.1.5. Extra-renal signs:

The ear, nose and throat (ENT) examination revealed erythematous angina in 8 patients, seromucosal otitis in 2 patients and cervical adenopathy in 3 patients.

There was no purpura or other specific lesion on skin examination in any of our patients.

The rest of the abdominal, neurological and joint examinations were unremarkable.

2.3. Biological check-up :

2.3.1. Renal function:

The mean urea was 13.54 ±11 mmol/1, with extremes ranging from 2.5 mmol/1 to 59 mmol/1.

Median creatinemia was 190 pmol/l with extremes between 30 pmol/l and 2013 pmol/l. Median clearance was 33.9 ml/min/1.73 m^2 SC [2-267.45 ml/min/1.73 m^2 SC], The breakdown of the population studied according to GFR is shown in Figure 9.

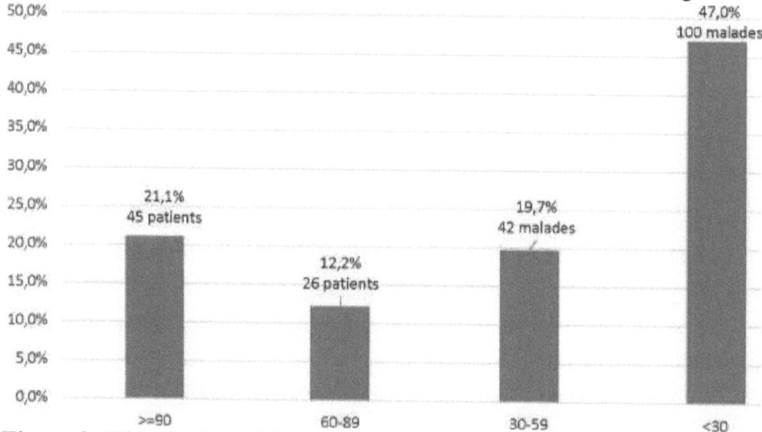

Figure 9: Distribution of the population studied according to glomerular filtration rate

2.3.2. Blood ionogram:

The median natremia was 138 mmol/1, with extremes between 118 and 146 mmol/1. The median kalemia was 4.5 mmol/1 with extremes between 2.7 and 7.1 mmol/1. At the time of hospitalisation, forty patients (18.7%) had hyperkalaemia and fifteen (7%) had hypokalaemia.

2.3.3. Phospho-calcium balance:

Mean calcemia was 2.28 mmol/1, with extremes ranging from 1.28 to 2.9 mmol/1. Initial hypocalcemia was observed in 39% of patients. Hypercalcemia was present in only 3 patients.

Mean phosphatemia was 1.48 mmol/1, with extremes between 0.6 and 4.75 mmol/1. The median alkaline phosphatase was 78 mmol/1, with values ranging from 29 to 579 mmol/1. Elies were elevated in 38 patients (17.8%).

2.3.4. 24-hour laproteinuria :

The median 24h proteinuria was 2.6 g/24h with extremes ranging from 0 to 46.17 g/24h. Nephrotic proteinuria (>3g/24h) was observed in 98 patients (46%).

The distribution of patients according to 24-hour proteinuria was as follows:

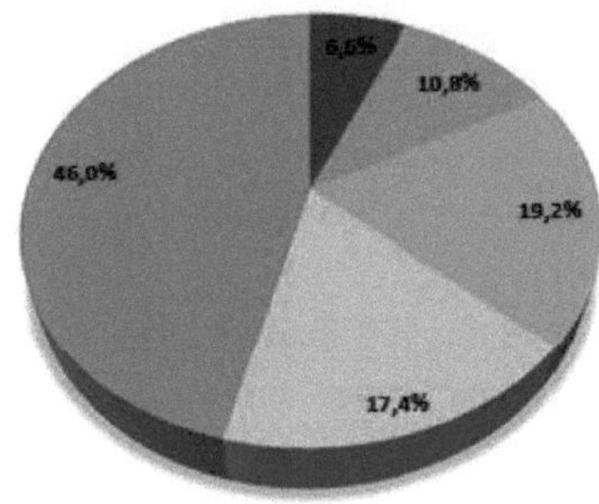

Figure 10: Distribution of patients according to twenty-four hour proteinuria value

2.3.5. Plasma protein electrophoresis:

Plasma protein electrophoresis was performed in 169 patients.

The average protein level was 63.92 ± 10.51 g/1 with extremes ranging from 32 a 90 g/1.

Mean albuminemia was 33.9 ± 8.7 g/1 with extremes ranging from 5.8 to 55g/l.

Mean alpha 1 globulin was 2.57 ± 1.73 g/1 with extremes between 1.2 and 17g/l.

Mean alpha 2 globulin was 9.1 ± 2.5 g/1 with extremes between 4 and 23,3 g/1.

The mean beta globulin was 8.97 ± 2.27 g/1, with extremes between 4 and 8 g/1. 19,1 g/1.

The mean gamma globulin was 9.92 ± 3.47 g/1, with extremes between 2.1 and 20 g/1. A nephrotic syndrome was found in 45 cases (21%). The impurities of the nephrotic syndrome are summarised in Table IX.

Table IX: Impurities in the nephrotic syndrome

SN impurity	Workforce	Percentage (%)
HTA	0	0
Hm	6	13,3
IR	2	4,4
HTA+IR	5	11,1
Hm + IR	5	11,1
Hm + HTA	6	13,3
HTA + IR + Hm	18	40

Hm: hematuria; HTA: arterial hypertension; IR: organic renal failure; NS: nephrotic syndrome

2.3.6. Themogram study:

The mean haemoglobin level was 11.34 ± 2.54 g/dl [5-18.5 g/dl], normocytic normochromic anaemia was observed in 116 patients (54.4%).

The mean white blood cell count was 7502 elements/mm^3 with extremes ranging from 3400 to 19800 elements/mm^3 . Hyperleukocytosis was noted in 26 patients (12.2%).

Platelets averaged 251,018 elements/mm^3 with extremes ranging from 127,000 to 646,000 elements/mm^3 . Nine patients had thrombocytopenia.

2.3.7. Lipid profile:

Cholesterolemia was measured in 187 patients. The mean value was 5.48 ± 2.07 mmol/1 [3-15.48 mmol/1]. Hypercholesterolemia was observed in 70 patients (37.4%). Triglyceride levels were measured in 189 patients. The mean value was 1.87 ± 0.98 mmol/1 [0.26-6.4 mmol/1]. Forty-seven patients had hypertriglyceridemia (24.8%).

2.3.8. Uricemia:

Mean uricemia was 428 mmol/1, with extremes ranging from 280 to 741 mmol/1. Hyperuricemia was observed at the time of diagnosis in 42% of cases.

2.3.9. Liver function tests:

On average, aspartate aminotransferase (ASAT) was equal to 6 IU/1 and alanine aminotransferase (ALAT) to 4 IU/1. Two patients had hepatic cytolysis at 7 and 10 times normal. No cause for this cytolysis was identified.

The median gamma-glutamyl-transpeptidase (GGT) level was 20 IU/1, with extremes ranging from 5 to 361 IU/1.

Mean total bilirubinemia was 8.1 mmol/1.

2.3.10. Immunological tests:

2.3.10.1. Serum IgA:

Serum IgA was measured in 77 patients. They were increased in 6 cases (7.8%).

2.3.10.2. The complementser:

The C3 and C4 fractions of the serum complement were measured in 97 patients. C3 was consumed by seven patients (7.2%), while C4 was consumed by two patients (2.1%).

The CH50 hemolytic complement assay was performed in 88 cases. It was reduced in 12 cases (13.6%).

2.3.10.3. Anti-nuclear antibodies:

Anti-nuclear antibodies were measured in 107 patients and were positive in 6. Anti-DNA was negative in all patients.

2.4. Radiological examinations :

2.4.1. Renal ultrasound:

All patients underwent renal ultrasound. The mean kidney size was 10.18 cm on the right and 10.44 cm on the left. Kidney size was reduced in 42 cases (19.7%). Eighty-one patients (38%) had cortico-sinus dedifferentiation.

2.4.2. Chest X-ray:

Chest X-rays were taken in 131 patients and showed :

- Cardiomegaly in 6 patients.
- Pulmonary overload in 12 cases.
- Interstitial syndrome in 2 patients.
- Elie was normal in the rest of the patients.

2.4.3. Cardiac ultrasound:

Cardiac ultrasound (CUS) was performed in 40 patients as part of the work-up for hypertension or as part of the pre-EER work-up. Pericardial effusion was found in 6 cases (15%). Left ventricular ejection fraction was reduced in 3 cases (7.5%).

2.5. Anatomopathological study :

After eliminating contraindications, ultrasound-guided percutaneous renal biopsy (PRB) was performed in 211 patients. Two patients underwent CT-guided RBB (due to the presence of renal cysts).

2.5.1. DelaidelaPBR:

The median time between PBR and the onset of the disease was 51 days, with extremes ranging from 2 to 1460 days.

2.5.2. Indications for renal biopsy:

The indications for PBR in our study are summarised in Table X.

Table X: Indications for renal biopsy in our population

Indications	*Number*	*Percentage (%)*
HU isolated	*4*	1,9
Isolated IR	*0*	0
IR with HU without proteinuria	2	0,9
Ptu24h between]0- 0.5g/24h[	8	3,8
Ptu24h between [0.5-3g/24h[.	101	47,4
Ptu24h > 3g/24h without SN	53	24,9
SN	45	21,1

HU: hematuria; IR: renal failure; Ptu24h: twenty-four hour proteinuria; SN: nephrotic syndrome.

2.5.3. Indications for the secondPBR :

Nine patients (4.2%) had two renal biopsies. The indications for the second PBR are summarised in Figure 11.

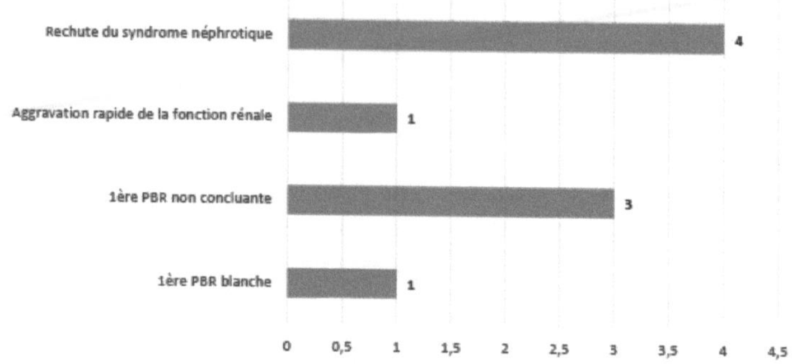

Figure 11: Indications for a second renal biopsy

2.5.4. Complications of renal biopsy:

Twenty-one patients developed a post-PBR complication (9.9%).

Four had transient macroscopic haematuria (19%). Only one PBR was complicated by an arteriovenous fistula. Sixteen patients had peri-renal hematomas (76.2%), with deglobulation in four patients, three of whom required transfusion. All hematomas healed spontaneously.

2.5.5. Optical microscopic study:

We have divided the lesions observed according to their sector: glomerular, tubulointerstitial and vascular.

2.5.5.1. Glomerular lesions:

The median number of glomeruli was 8 [2-65].

The median number of permeable glomeruli was 10 [0-55] and the number of sclerotic glomeruli (in sealing loaf) was 5 [0-38].

The lesions observed in permeable glomeruli are summarised in Table XI.

Table XI: Glomerular lesions in our population

Glomerular lesions	*Frequency*	*Percentage (%)*
Mesangial thickening	144	67,6
Mesangial proliferation	136	63,8
Segmental glomerulosclerosis	152	71,4
Endo-capillary proliferation	18	8,5
Podocytosis	89	41,8
Fibrinoid necrosis	12	5,6
Extra-capillary proliferation	36	16,9

- Mesangial proliferation: This was noted in 136 patients (63.8%). It was minimal in 37 biopsies, moderate in 80 biopsies and severe in 19 biopsies.
- Glomerulosclerosis: Segmental glomerulosclerosis was observed in 152 patients (71.4%). Thirteen patients (8.5%) had global glomerulosclerosis.
- Extra-capillary proliferation: thirty-six patients (16.9%) had extra-capillary

proliferation. The crescents were cellular in 14 biopsies, fibrocellular in 22 biopsies and fibrous in 15 biopsies.

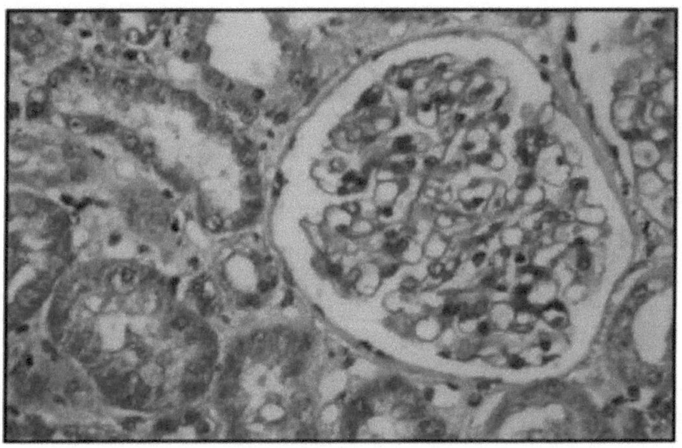

Photo 1: Optically normal kidney (M0E0S0T0C0)
Masson trichrome, magnification* x *400

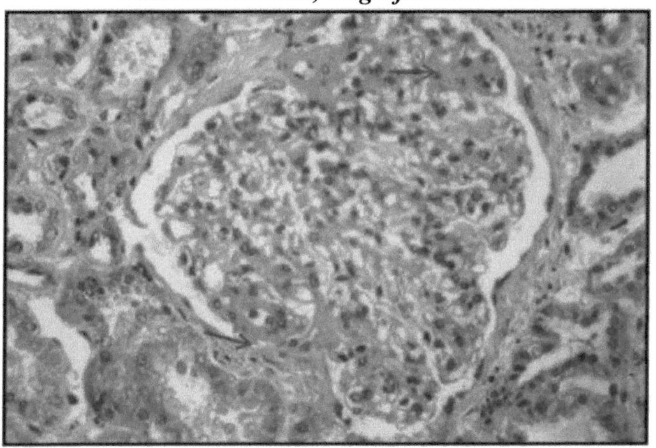

Photo 2 : Mesangial thickening with mesangial proliferation
(→)
and flocculo-capsular accolement (→)
Masson trichrome, magnification *400

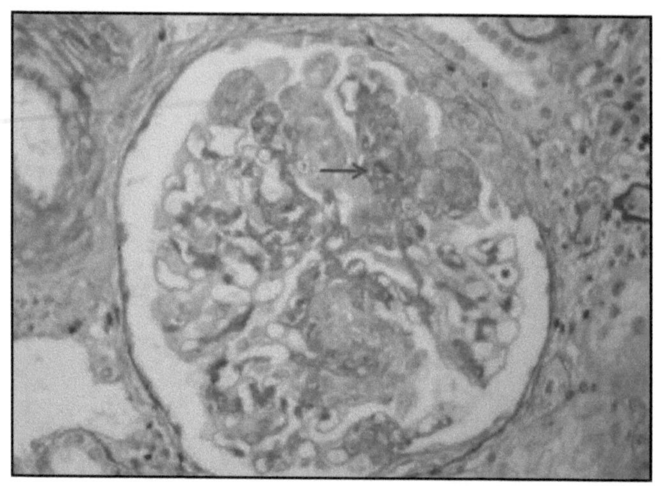

Photo 3: Endo-capillary proliferation at PAS, magnification *400

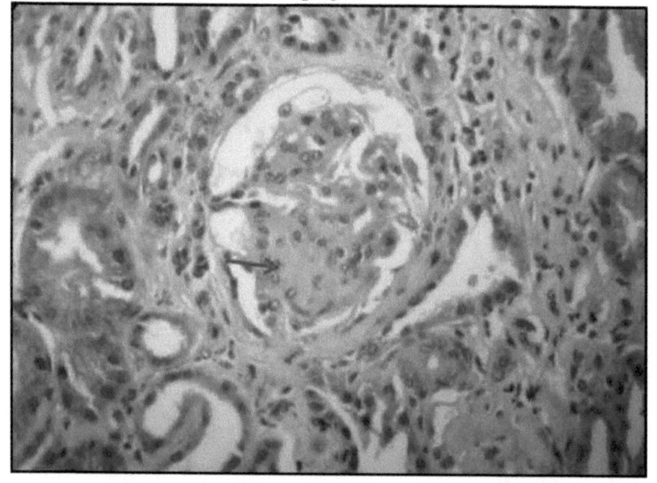

Photo 4: Segmental glomerulosclerosis Masson trichrome, magnification *200

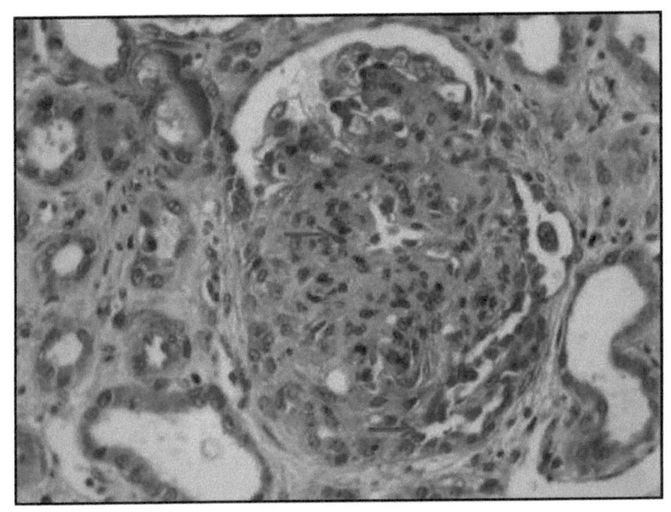

Photo 5: Mesangial proliferation (→) with cell crescent
()→
Masson trichrome, magnification *400

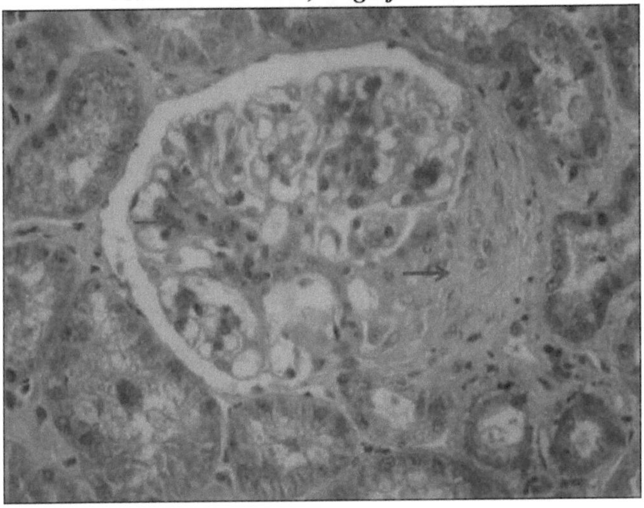

Photo 6: Mesangial proliferation (→) with fibro-cellular crescent ( )→
Masson trichrome, magnification x 400

2.5.5.2. Tubulointerstitial lesions:

An interstitial inflammatory infiltrate was noted in 116 biopsies (54%). It consisted mainly of mononuclear cells.

Tubular necrosis was observed in 9% of cases.

Interstitial fibrosis and/or tubular atrophy was detected in 155 biopsies (72.8%).

We noted the presence of cylinders in 70% of biopsies. They were exclusively hyaline in 73 biopsies and hematic in 24 biopsies. A combination of hematic and hyaline cylinders was observed in 43 biopsies. The combination of three types of cylinders (hyaline, hematic, granular) was noted in seven biopsies.

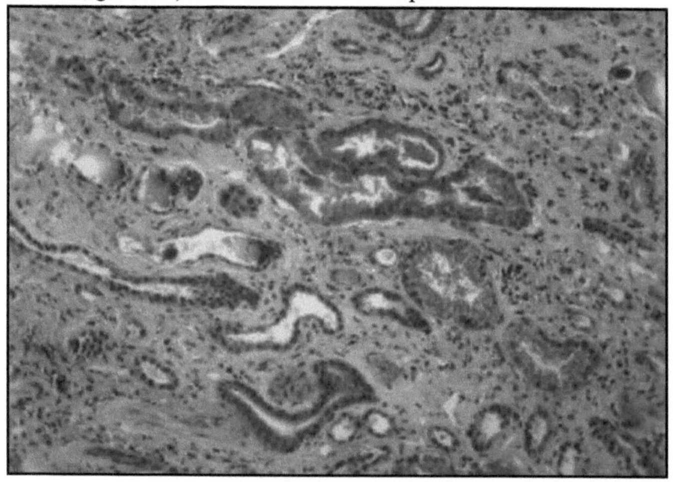

Photo 7: Interstitial fibrosis/tubular atrophy
Masson trichrome, magnification* x *400

2.5.5.3. Vascular lesions:

Vascular involvement such as arteriosclerosis was found in 61 patients (28.6%). We noted the presence of arteriosclerosis lesions in 90 biopsies (42.2%).

Thrombotic microangiopathy (TMA) lesions were present in 32% of cases.

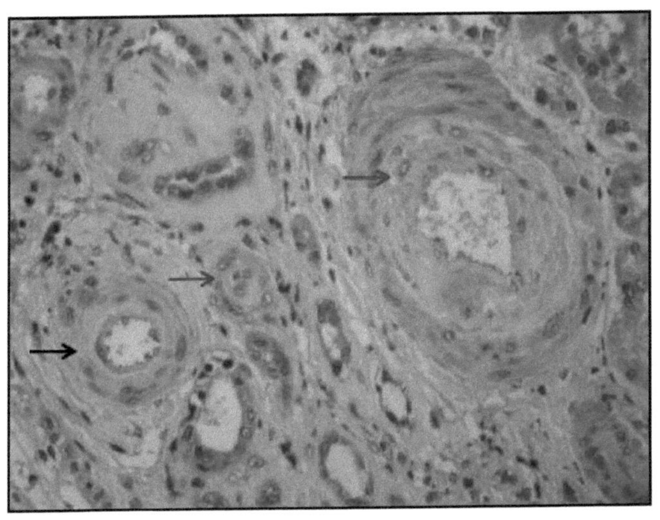

Photo 8: Arteriosclerosis →) -
thrombotic microangiopthia
(→) - arteriosclerosis ( )→
Masson trichrome, magnification x 200

2.5.6. Oxford classification:

The two most common histological lesions were segmental glomerulosclerosis (SI) (71.4%) and mesangial proliferation (Ml) (63.8%).
The distribution of the different histological lesions according to the Oxford MEST-C classification is shown in Table XII.

Table XII: Breakdown of patients according to the Oxford MEST-C classification

Optical microscopy data		*Frequency*	*Percentage (%)*
Proliferation	MO	77	36,2
mesangial (M)	Ml	136	63,8
Proliferation	E0	195	91,5
endocapillary(E)	El	18	8,5
Glomerulosclerosis	SO	61	28,6
segmental (S)	SI	152	71,4
Atrophy	TO	58	27,2
Tubular/Fibrosis	T1	72	33,8
interstitial (T)	T2	83	39
Cellular crescents	CO	177	83,1
/Fibro-cellular (C)	C1-C2	36	16,9

The median cumulative Oxford score was 3 [0-6].

2.5.7. Direct immunofluorescence study:

In all cases, Elie showed diffuse and predominant mesangial fixation of anti-IgA sera. Anti IgM was positive in 63.8% of cases and anti-IgG in 16%. The sites were mesangial and segmental. Mesangial C3 complement fixation was observed in 180 patients (84.5%). Clq fixation was noted in 8.4% of biopsies.

Binding of kappa and lambda light chains was investigated in 119 patients. Mesangial binding of these chains was observed in 80% of cases, with a predominance of lambda light chains.

The distribution of the different types of immunoglobulin deposits is shown in Figure 12.

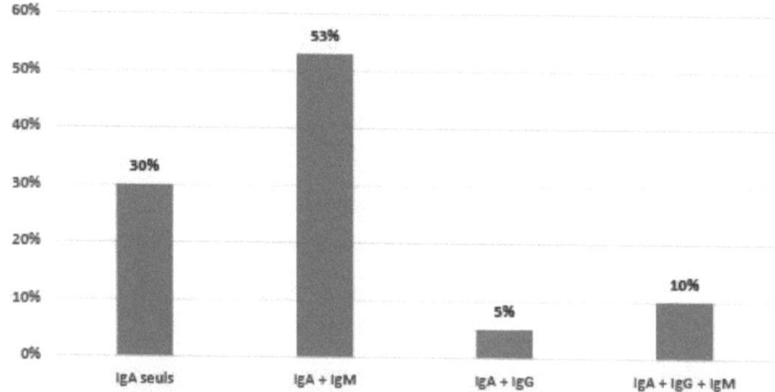

Figure 12: Distribution of different types of immunoglobulin deposits in our population

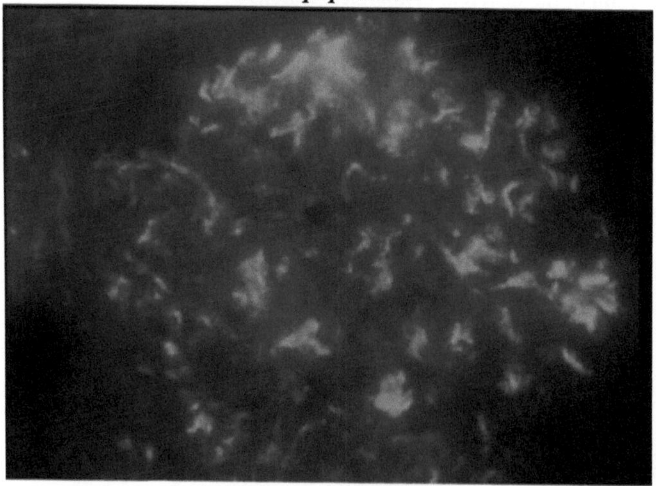

Photo 9: Mesangial deposits of immunoglobulin A in immunofluorescence

2.5.8. Electron microscopy study :

Biopsies from three patients were examined by electron microscopy. We noted diffuse mesangial lgA deposition and effacement of podocyte pedicels in all biopsies. This effacement was diffuse in two cases and segmental in the third biopsy.

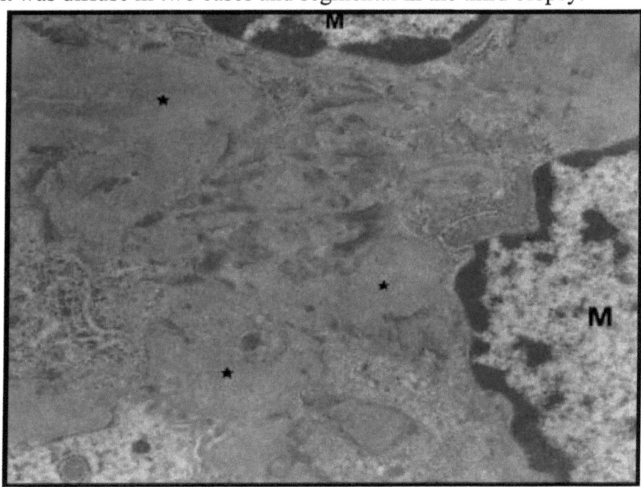

Photo 10: Measured immunoglobulin A deposits by electron microscopy

2.6. Therapeutic management :

2.6.1. Conservative treatment:

Conservative treatment included:

- **Smoking cessation :**

Smoking cessation was achieved in 34 patients, corresponding to 39.1% of smokers.

- **Fluid restriction:**

Hydrosode restriction was not systematically reported in the files.

- **Lipid-lowering treatment:**

Thirty-eight patients had rccu lipid-lowering treatment (17.8%). These were statins in twenty-nine cases (76.3%) and fibrates in nine cases (23.7%).

- **Treatment of hyperuricemia :**

Twenty-six patients (12.2%) were started on Allopurinol.

- **Antihypertensive and nephroprotective treatment :**

A total of 121 patients (56.8%) received renin angiotensin aldosterone system inhibitors (RAASI).

Thirty-seven (30.5%) normotensive patients were started on a low dose of BSRAA for anti-proteinuric purposes.

The different classes of antihypertensive drugs used are summarised in table XIII.

Table XIII: Classes of antihypertensives

Class	*Frequency*	*Percentage*

BSRAAIEC	100	46,9
ARAII	21	9,9
Calcium inhibitor	123	57,7
Diuretics	50	23,4
Central antihypertensive	40	18,8
Alpha bioquant	7	3,3
Beta bioquant	73	34,3

BSRAA: renin angiotensin aldosterone system blockers; ACE inhibitors: ACE inhibitors; ARBs: angiotensin II receptor antagonists.

The converting enzyme inhibitors used were Captopril in 86 patients, Enalapril in seven patients, Ramipril in five patients and Perindopril in two patients.

The angiotensin II receptor antagonists present were: Irbesartan in 14 patients, Losartan in four patients, Valsartan in one patient, Telmisartan in one patient and Candesartan in one patient.

Patients had rccи antihypertensive monotherapy, bitherapy, tritherapy, quadritherapy in 27%, 20% ,23%,8% of cases respectively.

- **Tonsillectomy and fish oil:**

Tonsillectomy was performed in 5 cases (2.3%). No patient received fish oil.

- **Antibiotic treatment :**

Antibiotic treatment was present in 44 patients (20.7%). It was indicated for the treatment of angina (25%), bronchopulmonary infections (31.9%), urinary tract infections (20.4%), dental infections (9.1%), skin infections (11.4%) and endovascular portal infections (2.2%).

The average prescription period was one day [0-15 days],

The classes of antibiotics used are detailed in Figure 13.

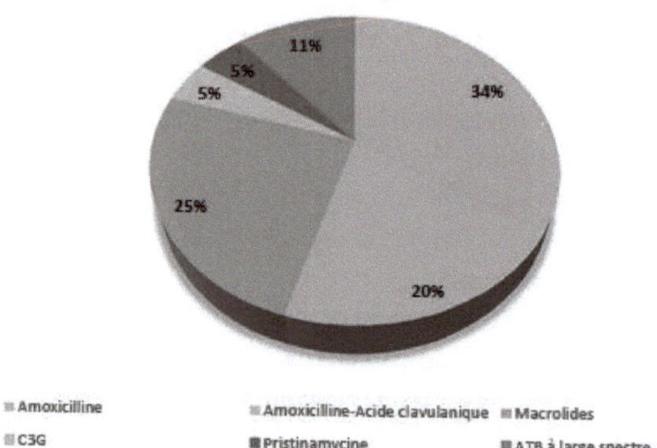

Figure 13: Classes of antibiotics used in our patients during hospitalisation

2.6.2. Immunosuppressive treatment:

2.6.2.1. Corticosteroid treatment:

Corticosteroid treatment was present in 91 patients (42.7%). The indications were distributed as follows: (Figure 14)

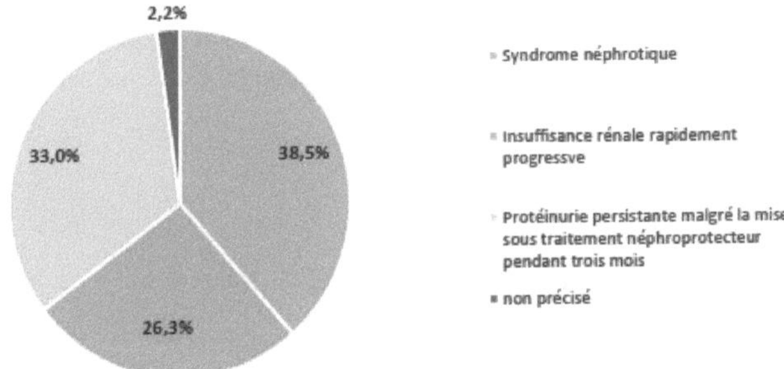

Figure 14: Distribution of patients by indication for corticosteroid therapy In these patients, the median GFR was 26 ml/min/1.73 m^2 SC
[3 - 267 ml/min/1.73 m^2 SC] and median proteinuria was 3.5g/24h.
[0.67 -46.17 g/24h],
Two treatment plans have been adopted:

- Fifty-four patients (59.3%) were rccи oral corticotherapie at a dose of lmg/Kg/d for one month followed by a gradual taper.
- Thirty-seven patients (40.7%) were placed on the Pozzi Protocol.

2.6.2.2. Cyclophosphamide:

It was present in 2 patients in association with corticoids and nephroprotective treatment.

o The first patient was 30 years old, with no previous medical history and a drug addiction. He presented with rapidly progressive glomerulonephritis and severe hypertension. Initial GFR was 17.51 ml/min/l,73m^2 SC. 24-hour proteinuria was 4.01 g/24h. The immunological work-up was without abnormalities. Histological lesions were severe. We noted 50% sclerotic glomeruli, extra-capillary proliferation, hematic, granular cylinders and MAT lesions. The PBR was classified as M1E1S0T2C1. With nephroprotective treatment, the patient received prednisone at a dose of lmg/kg/d and 2 boluses of cyclophosphamide 500 mg at 2-week intervals. Given the rapid progression to end-stage renal failure, the cyclophosphamide was stopped.

o The second patient was a young man aged 18, from a first-degree consanguineous marriage, with a history of recurrent macroscopic hematuria concomitant with ENT infections. His nephropathy was revealed by an impure nephrotic syndrome caused by hematuria and renal failure. A first PBR showed endo and extra capillary proliferation. The patient was put on nephroprotective treatment, corticoids and cyclophosphamide, with remission of the nephrotic syndrome. The course was marked by frequent relapses over 5 years. A second PBR was carried out, showing a worsening of the tubular lesions. Terminal stage was reached after 73 months.

2.6.2.3. Mycophenolate mofetil (MMF) :

MMF was used in three patients with cortico-dependent nephrotic syndrome. The prescribed dose was 2g/d.

2.6.2.4. *Cyclosporine:*

Elie was prescribed to a single patient for a cortico-resistant nephrotic syndrome. The distribution of patients according to the treatment chosen is shown in Figure 15.

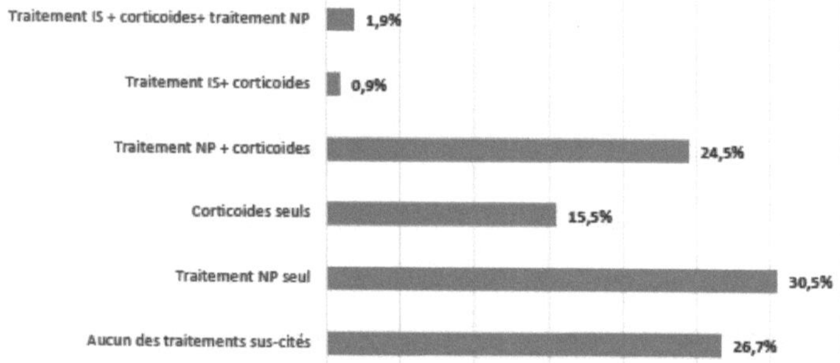

Figure 15: Breakdown of patients by type of treatment received

2.7. Evolution :

2.7.1. Follow-up time:

The median follow-up time in our study was 24 months, with extremes ranging from 1 to 360 months. Eighty-five patients (40%) were followed for less than one year.

2.7.2. Evolution of arterial pressure:

After 3 months, median SBP was 130 mmHg [100-180 mmHg] and median DBP was 80 mmHg [60-110 mmHg],

At the end of follow-up, the median PAS was 130 mmHg, with extremes between 100 and 190 mmHg, while the median DBP was 80 mmHg, with extremes ranging from 50 to 20 mmHg.

2.7.3. Evolution of Proteinuria and Thematuria:

After 3 months, the median 24-hour proteinuria was 1g/24h, with extremes ranging from 0 to 12g/24h.

At the end of follow-up, median proteinuria was 0.51g/24h, with extremes ranging from 0 to 17.7g/24h.

The median hematuria was one cross at 3 months and at the end of follow-up.

Changes in proteinuria and haematuria during the study period are shown in Table XV.

Table XIV: Changes in proteinuria and thematuria during follow-up

Deadline	*Median Pu24h (g/24h)*	*Median hematuria (cross)*
1 month	1,3 (0-19,5)	1(0-3)
3 months	1 (0 -12)	1(0-3)
6 months	0,7 (0 - 7,5)	1(0-3)
1 year	0,57 (0 - 8,6)	1(0-3)
18 months	0,75 (0-11)	1(0-3)

2 years	0,95 (0 - 12)	1(0-3)
End of monitoring	0,51 (0-17,7)	1(0-3)

Pu24h: twenty-four-hour protein shortage

2.7.4. Evolution of renal function:

2.7.4.1. Chronic kidney disease:

At the end of follow-up, median urea was 8.5 mmol/1 with extremes ranging from 2.8 to 45 mmol/1. The median creatinemia was 161 pmol/l with extremes ranging from 46 to 1220 pmol/l.

Changes in renal function during the follow-up period are shown in Table XVI.

Table XV: Changes in renal function during follow-up

Deadline	Median uree (mmol/l)	Median creatinemia (pmol/l)
1 month	7,8 (2,5 - 42,8)	141 (40-617)
3 months	6,9 (2,4 - 35,8)	146 (47 - 527)
6 months	6,55 (2,5-35)	109 (45 - 522)
1 year	7,4 (2-41)	118 (45 - 1220)
18 months	7,4 (0,5 - 44)	137 (44- 1331)
2 years	7,35 (3,1 -45)	124 (41 - 1102)
End of monitoring	8,5 (2,8 - 45)	161 (46- 1220)

At the end of follow-up, the distribution of patients by stage of chronic kidney disease was as follows (Figure 16)

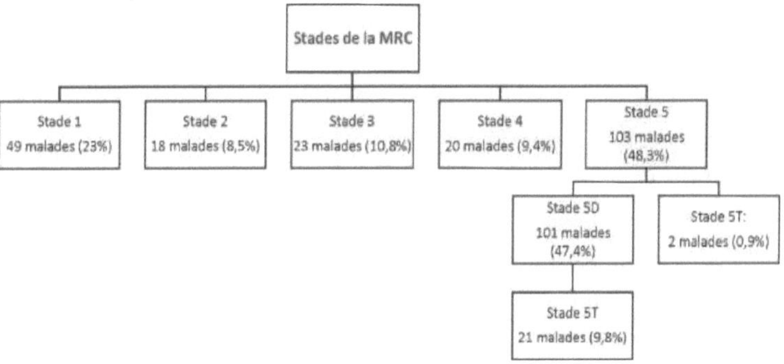

CKD: Chronic kidney disease; 5D: Patients with dialysis CKD; 5T: Patients with transplant CKD

Figure 16: Breakdown of the population studied by stage of chronic kidney disease at the time of the latest news

1.7.4.2. Terminal stage:

End stage was reached in 103 patients (48.3%). The median time from diagnosis of IgA nephropathy to the need for EER was 7 months, with extremes ranging from 0 (acute dialysis) to 226 months.

The modalities of extra-renal purification were: hemodialysis (HD) in 83 patients (80.5%) and peritoneal dialysis (PD) in 18 patients (17.4%). Four patients were initially on PD but were transferred to HD because of recurrent peritonitis. Two patients underwent pre-emptive renal transplantation without recourse to EBRT (0.1%).

1.7.4.3. Renal transplantation:

In our population, 23 patients (10.8%) had undergone renal transplantation (RT). Two patients (0.1%) underwent preemptive renal transplantation. RT was performed from a living donor kidney in 18 cases (78.3%) and from a cadaveric kidney in 5 cases (21.7%). The mean time between RT and the start of extra-renal purification was 3 years, with extremes ranging from 0 to 100 years.

The characteristics of renal transplant patients are summarised in Table XVII.

Table XVI: Characteristics of renal transplant patients

Features	*Number*
Total number of transplant patients	23
Cadaveric donor	5
Living donor	18 including 2 pre-emptive
HLA identity number :	
No	2
A single	1
Two	2
Three	13
Four	5
Induction treatment: Thymoglobulins	23
Maintenance treatment :	
Ciclosporin-MMF-Solupred	7
Prograf-MMF-Solupred	13
Ciclosporin-Imurel-Solupred	2
Rapamune-MMF-Solupred	1
Average follow-up time (years)	8
Graft survival	
A lan	22
At 2 years	20
At 5 years	18
Recurrence of IgA nephropathy	6

HLA: major histocompatibility complex; MMF: mycophenolate mofetil; TR: renal transplantation

Only one patient had experienced acute rejection due to graft artery thrombus resulting in total graft ischemia and same day detransplantation. The patient had been transplanted from an apparent living donor with 0 HLA identity.

Thirteen patients (56.5%) underwent graft biopsy. PBG was performed in 11 patients for worsening graft function and in 2 patients to investigate isolated proteinuria.

PBG results were as follows: lesions related to anticalcineurin toxicity in 4 biopsies and acute cell rejection in 3 biopsies.

LgA deposits were objective in eight patients, six of whom had associated histological lesions. The mean time to recurrence was 8 years, with extremes ranging from 3 to 6 years.

2.7.5. Evolving complications:

2.7.5.1. Cortico-induced diabetes:

Cortico-induced diabetes was observed in 10 patients (11%) after long-term corticotherapy.

2.7.5.2. Infectious complications:

Twenty-six patients (26.8%) developed infectious complications following corticosteroid and immunosuppressive treatment. The most frequent infections were: digestive tract infections (8 patients), pneumonia (2 patients), recurrent urinary tract infections (3 patients), bacterial skin infections (6 patients), herpes zoster (3 patients) and viral hepatitis (4 patients).

2.7.5.3. Neoplasia:

The neoplastic complications observed were:

- Invasive ductal carcinoma of the breast (2 cases).
- An intracranial expansive process (1 case).

With a median onset delay of 3 years [12-16 years].

2.7.6.Deaths:

Two deaths occurred (0.9%) during the study period:

- A 36-year-old patient died with an altered neurological state related to an intracranial expansive process occurring 15 years after renal transplantation.
- A 16-year-old female patient was admitted to hospital for the management of rapidly progressive renal failure associated with IgA nephropathy. Elie was put on corticotherapie with recourse to hemodialysis. Elie died following a state of septic shock with an endovascular origin, despite appropriate antibiotic therapy.

3. ANALYTICAL STUDY :

3.1. Anatomical-clinical correlations :

3.1.1. Correlations between mesangial proliferation (Ml) and clinical-biological data:

Mesangial proliferation (Ml) was correlated with the presence of hypertension (p=0.008) and renal failure (p=0.0045) at the time of diagnosis of nephropathy (Table XVIII).

Table XVII: Correlations between mesangial proliferation and the data clinico-biological

	MO	*MI*	*P*
Genre :			
H	32,35%	67,65%	0,19
F	42,8%	57,2%	
Age (Year)	35,7	33,8	0,3
Tobacco	33,3%	66,6%	0,37
CDD :			

HTA	26,8%	73,2%	**0,008***
HU macroscopic	38,6%	61,4%	0,78
SN	29,2%	70,8%	0,1
IR	31%	69%	**0,047***
PAS (mmHg)	146	150,3	0,34
DBP (mmHg)	87,6	89,6	0,43
GFR (ml/min/l,73m^2 SC)	55,34	46,65	0,17
PU24h(g/24h)	3,2	3,9	0,28
Uricemia(mmol/1)	387,2	430	0,054

M: male; F: female; CDD: circumstances of discovery; HTA: arterial hypertension; HU: hematuria; NS: nephrotic syndrome; IR: renal insufficiency; SAP: systolic blood pressure; DBP: diastolic blood pressure, GFR: glomerular filtration rate; Pu24H: 24-hour proteinuria; M: mesangial proliferation.

3.1.2. Correlations between endocapillary proliferation and clinical-biological data:

Endo-capillary proliferation (El) was correlated with age (p=0.021), smoking (p=0.027), the presence of initial renal failure (p=0.048) and hyperuricemia (p=0.029) with a statistically significant difference. (Table XIX).

Table XVIII: Correlations between endocapillary proliferations and clinico-biological data

	EO	*El*	*P*
Genre :			
H	89%	11%	0,07
F	96,1%	3,9%	
Age (Year)	33,9	41,1	**0,021***
Tobacco	86,2%	13,8%	**0,027***
CDD :			
HTA	88,9%	11,1%	0,28
HU macroscopic	95,5%	4,5%	0,35
SN	92,7%	87,5%	0,25
IR	87%	13%	**0,048***
PAS (mmHg)	148,2	154,2	0,42
DBP (mmHg)	88,4	90,7	0,7
GFR(ml/min/l,73m^2 SC)	50,6	36,9	0,2
PU24h(g/24h)	3,54	4,95	0,09
Uricemia(mmol/1)	407,5	495,9	**0,029***

M: male; F: female; CDD: circumstances of discovery; HU: haematuria; NS: nephrotic syndrome; IR: renal failure; SBP: systolic blood pressure; DBP: diastolic blood pressure, GFR: glomerular filtration rate; Pu24H: 24-hour proteinuria; E: endocapillary proliferation.

3.1.3. Correlations between segmental glomerulosclerosis and clinical-biological data:

Segmental glomerulosclerosis (SI) was correlated with the presence of initial renal failure (p<0.001), PAS (p=0.003), PAD (p=0.001) and hyperuricemia (p=0.003). (Table XX)

Table XIX: Correlations between segmental glomerulosclerosis and clinico-biological data

	SO	***SI***	***P***
Genre:			
H	27,2%	72,8%	0,32
F	31,2%	68,8%	
Age (Year)	33,5	34,9	0,48
Tobacco	24,1%	75,9%	0,22
CDD :			
HTA	17,6%	82,4%	**<0,001***
HU macroscopic	45,5%	54,6%	0,32
SN	33,3%	66,7%	0,47
IR	18,6%	71,4%	**<0,001***
PAS (mmHg)	137,8	153,1	**0,003***
DBP (mmHg)	81,8	91,7	**0,001***
GFR(ml/min/l,73m^2 SC)	74,5	39,9	**<0,001***
PU24h(g/24h)	3,86	3,58	0,68
Uricemia(mmol/1)	362,6	434,6	**0,003***

M: male; F: female; CDD: circumstances of discovery; HTA: arterial hypertension; HU: hematuria; IR: renal failure; NS: nephrotic syndrome; SAP: systolic blood pressure; DBP: diastolic blood pressure; GFR: glomerular filtration rate; Pu24H: 24-hour proteinuria; S: segmental glomerulosclerosis.

3.1.4. Correlations between tubular hypertrophy/interstitial flrosis and clinical-biological data:

Tubular atrophy/interstitial fibrosis (T1-T2) correlated with male sex (p=0.04), smoking (p=0.007) and the presence of hypertension indicative of nephropathy. Biologically, these lesions were correlated with the presence of a nephrotic syndrome, initial renal failure and hyperuricemia (p<0.001). On the other hand, the discovery of IgA nephropathy following an episode of macroscopic haematuria was associated with the absence of tubular atrophy/interstitial fibrosis on PBR, with a statistically significant difference (p=0.001) (Table XXI).

Table XX: Correlations between tubular muscular dystrophy/interstitial flrosis and

clinico-biological data

	TO	***Tl-2***	***P***
Genre :			
H	22,8%	77,2%	**0,04***
F	35,1%	63,9%	
Age	33	35	0,31
Tobacco	5,8%	94,2%	**0,007***

CDD :			
HTA	12,9%	87,1%	**<0,001***
HU macroscopic	54,5%	45,5%	**0,001[a]**
SN	45,8%	54,2%	**0,002***
IR	10,3%	89,7%	**<0,001***
PAS (mmHg)	129,5	156	**<0,001***
DBP (mmHg)	78,3	92,8	**<0,001***
GFR(ml/min/l,73m^2 SC)	94,31	33,13	**<0,001***
PU24h(g/24h)	4,34	3,37	0,12
Uricemia(mmol/1)	336,3	441,4	**<0,001***

M: male; F: female; CDD: circumstances of discovery; ATH: arterial hypertension. HU: hematuria; NS: nephrotic syndrome; IR: renal failure; SBP: systolic blood pressure; DBP: diastolic blood pressure; GFR: glomerular filtration rate; Pu24H: 24-hour proteinuria; T: tubular atrophy/interstitial fibrosis;[a] positive correlation.

3.1.5. Correlations between the presence of cellular/fibrocellular crescents and clinical-biological data:

The presence of crescents (C1-C2) was correlated with male sex (p=0.04), the presence of renal failure at the time of diagnosis (p=0.003) and low glomerular filtration rate (p=0.003) with a statistically significant difference (Table XXII).

Table XXI: Correlations between the presence of cell crescents/ fibrocellular and clinico-biological data

	CO	*Cl*	*P*
Genre :			
H	79,4%	20,6%	**0,04***
F	89,6%	10,4%	
Age (Year)	34,6	33,6	0,68
Tobacco	83,9%	82,5%	0,8
CDD :			
HTA	81,8%	76,6%	0,38
HU macroscopic	81,8%	83,6%	0,8
SN	83,3%	83%	1
IR	77,9%	94,1%	**0,003***
PAS (mmHg)	148,9	147,8	0,8
DBP (mmHg)	88,8	88,8	1
GFR(ml/min/l,73m^2 SC)	53,9	29,7	**0,003***
PU24h(g/l)	3,65	3,68	0,96
Uricemia(mmol/1)	407,1	453,9	0,07

M: male; F: female; CDD: circumstances of discovery; HTA: arterial hypertension; HU: hematuria; NS: nephrotic syndrome; IR: renal insufficiency; SAP: systolic blood pressure; DBP: diastolic blood pressure; GFR: glomerular filtration rate; Pu24H: 24-hour proteinuria; C: Croissants.

3.2. Risk factors for creatinemia doubling :

To study the revolution in renal function, we looked for risk factors for creatinemia doubling at 6 months.

Only high ADP values (p=0.04), the existence of initial renal failure (p=0.004) and the presence of Tl-2 tubular atrophy/interstitial fibrosis lesions on histology (p=0.02) were associated with a statistically significant risk of creatinemia doubling at 6 months (Table XXIII).

Table XXII: Clinical-biological, histological and therapeutic factors associated with creatinemia doubling at 6 months

Factors studied	*Doubling of creatinemia at 6 months*	*No doubling of creatinine at 6 months*	*P*
Genre :			
H	77%	61%	0,5
F	33%	38%	
Age (Year)	33,8	36,4	0,52
BMI $(kg/m)^2$	25,47	23,55	0,18
Tobacco	61,5%	37%	0,6
CDD :			
HU macroscopic	15,4%	27%	0,6
HTA	69,3%	46%	0,23
SN	15,4%	27%	0,35
IR	100%	62%	**0,004***
PAS (mmHg)	161	147	0,12
DBP (mmHg)	98,5	87,7	**0,04***
PU24h(g/24h)	3,43	4,63	0,12
Uricemia(mmol/1)	476	411	0,06
MEST-C score :			
M	Ml: 74.9	Ml: 59	0,17
E	El: 15.4%	El: 6% of sales	0,4
S	SI: 84.6	SI: 71	0,23
T	Tl-2: 100%.	Tl-2: 70%.	**0,02***
c	Cl-2: 15.4	Cl-2 :18	0,5
BSRAA	53,8%	72%	0,16
Corticoides	53,8%	60%	0,45

H: male; F: female; BMI: body mass index; CDD: circumstances of discovery; HU: hematuria; ATH: arterial hypertension, NS: nephrotic syndrome; IR: renal insufficiency; SBP: systolic blood pressure; DBP: diastolic blood pressure, GFR : glomerular filtration rate; Pu24H: 24-hour proteinuria; M: mesangial proliferation; E: endocapillary proliferation; S: segmental glomerulosclerosis; T: tubular atrophy/interstitial fibrosis; C: crescents; BSRAA: renin angiotensin aldosterone system blockers.

3.3. Risk factors for progression to the terminal stage:

3.3.1. Univariate study:

Renal survival without progression to CKD was estimated at 83.3% at 1 month, 74.3% at 6 months, 67.2% at 1 year and 62.9% at 2 years (Figure 17).

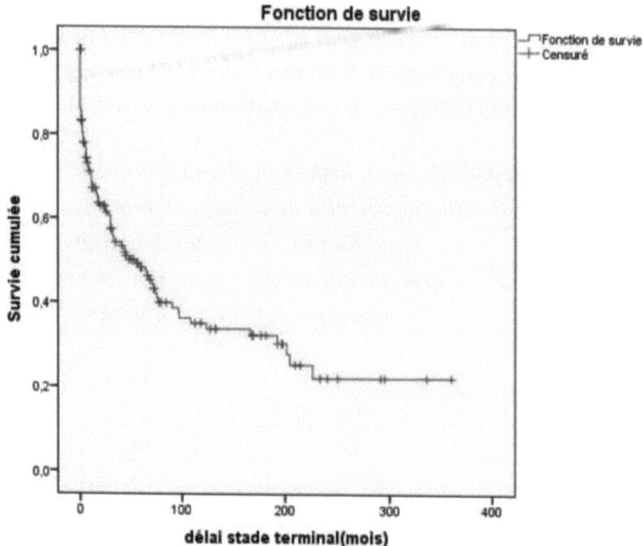

Figure 17: Renal survival of our population

In this univariate study, the following elements were associated with a higher risk of extra-renal cleansing:

- **Male sex (p=0.03)**
- **Advancing age (p=0.049)**
- **Smoking (p=0.012)**
- **Presence of renal failure (p<0.001) and arterial hypertension (p<0.001) at the time of diagnosis.**
- **Proteinuria >2 g/24 (p<0.001)**
- **Hyperuricemia (p=0.003)**
- **The presence of SI (p<0.001), Tl-2 (p<0.001) and Cl-2 (p=0.006) lesions at the PBR.**

On the other hand, the discovery of IgA nephropathy following an episode of macroscopic hematuria (p<0.001) or incidentally (by urine sediment anomaly) (p<0.001) and the use of BSRAA (p=0.032) were protective factors against progression to the terminal stage.

a) Epidemiological and clinical prognostic factors :

Male gender was associated with a poor renal prognosis, with a statistically significant difference (p=0.012) (Figure 18).

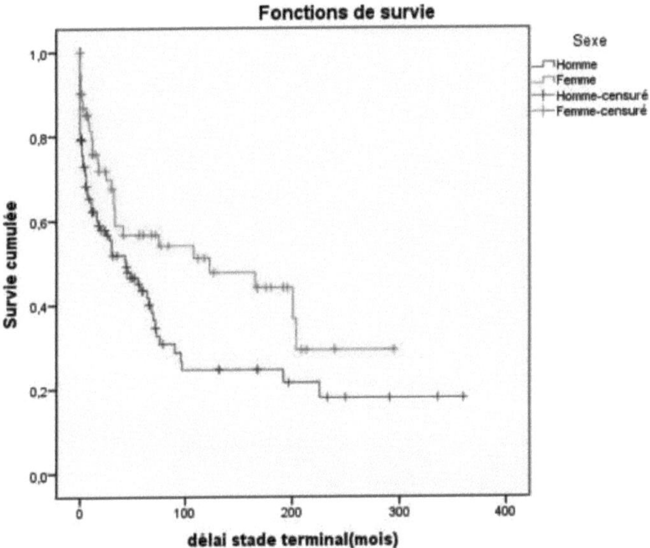

Figure 18: Kidney survival by gender

Smoking has a negative influence on renal prognosis (p=0.012) (figure 19).

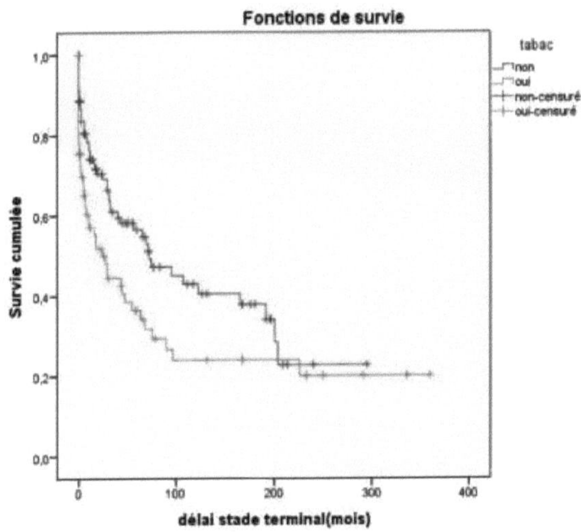

Figure 19: Kidney survival as a function of smoking habits

Renal survival was better for patients whose nephropathy was revealed by macroscopic hematuria (p>0.001) (Figure 20).

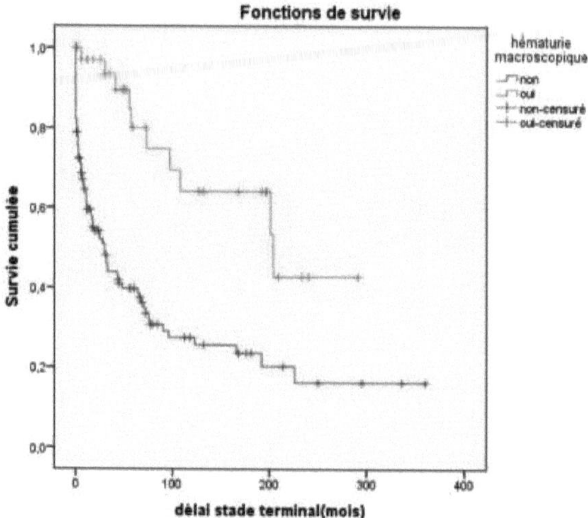

Figure 20: Kidney survival as a function of initial macroscopic hematuria

The presence of hypertension at the time of NIgA diagnosis had a significant impact on renal survival (p<0.001) (Figure 21).

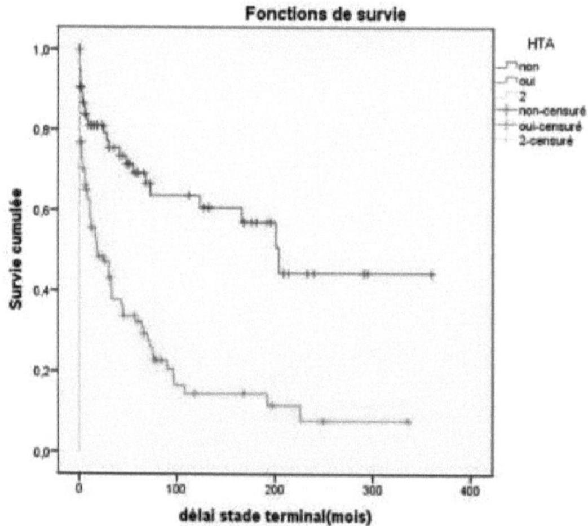

Figure 21: Renal survival as a function of [hypertension

Renal survival was better in cases of incidental detection of nephropathy during routine urinalysis (p<0.001) (Figure 22).

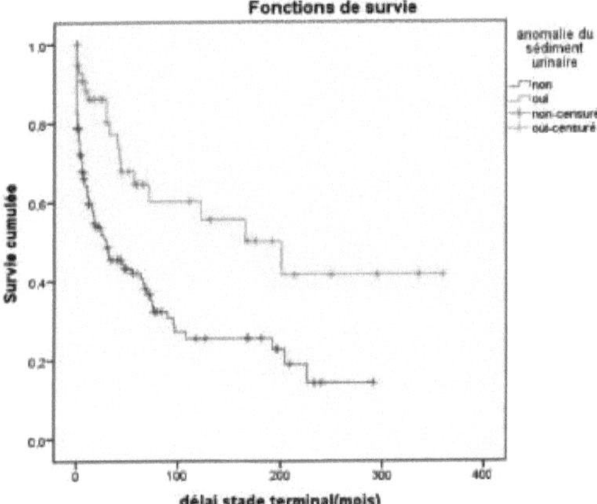

Figure 22: Kidney survival as a function of urine sediment anomalies

b) Biological prognostic factors :

The presence of renal failure at the time of diagnosis had a significant impact on renal survival ($p<0.001$) (Figure 23).

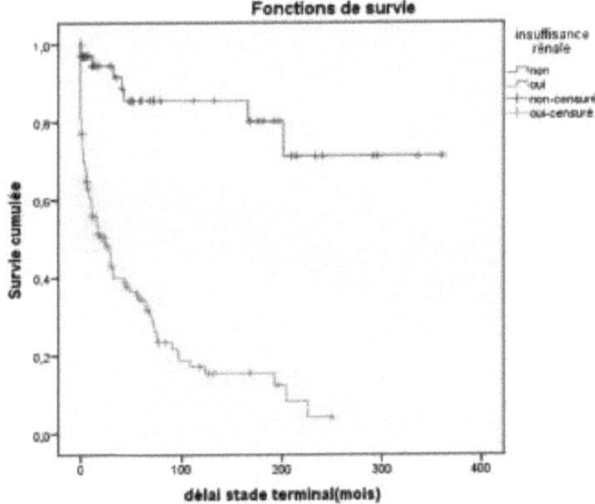

Figure 23: Renal survival as a function of the presence of initial renal failure

Proteinuria >2 g/24 hours was associated with a poor renal prognosis ($p<0.001$) (Figure 24).

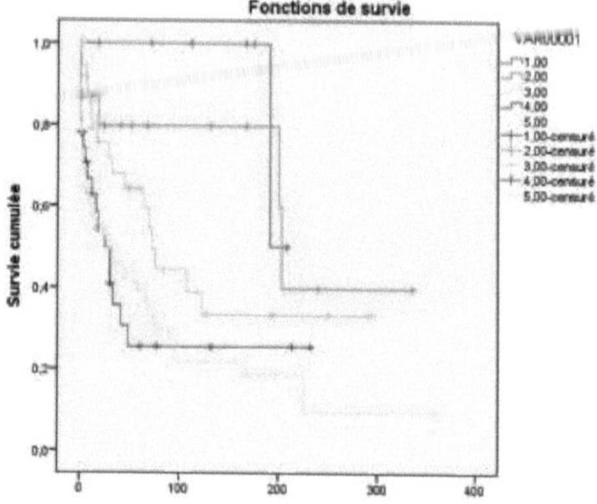

time to final stage(months)

Figure 24: Renal survival as a function of twenty-four hour proteinuria

Hyperuricemia was associated with poor renal prognosis with a significant difference (p=0.003) (Figure 25).

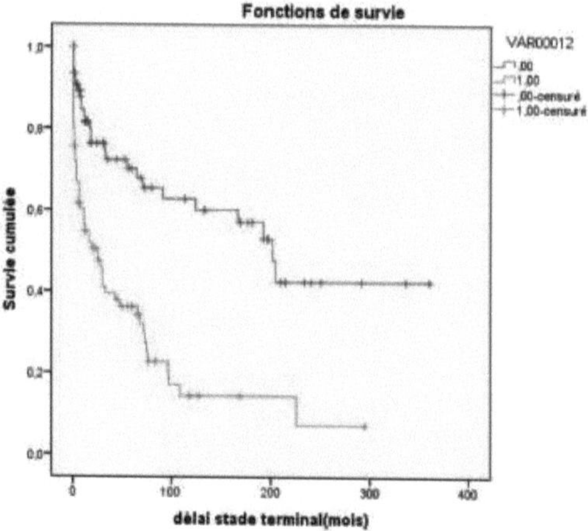

Figure 25: Renal survival as a function of hyperuricemia

c) Histological prognostic factors :

The presence of SI (p<0.001), Tl-2 (p<0.001) and Cl-2 (p=0.006) lesions on renal biopsy had a significant impact on renal survival (Figure 26).

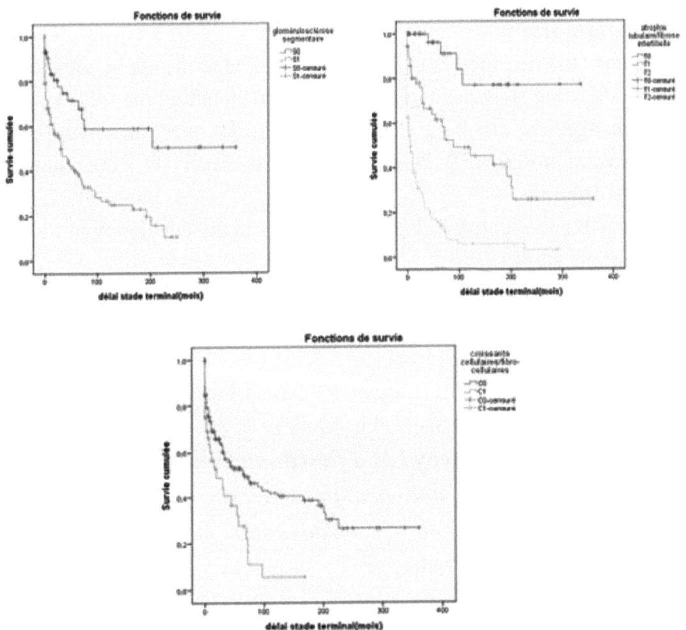

Figure 26: Renal survival as a function of MEST-C classification score oxford

d) Therapeutic prognostic factors :

Survival was better when nephroprotective treatment with renin angiotensin aldosterone system blockers was administered (p=0.032) (Figure 27).

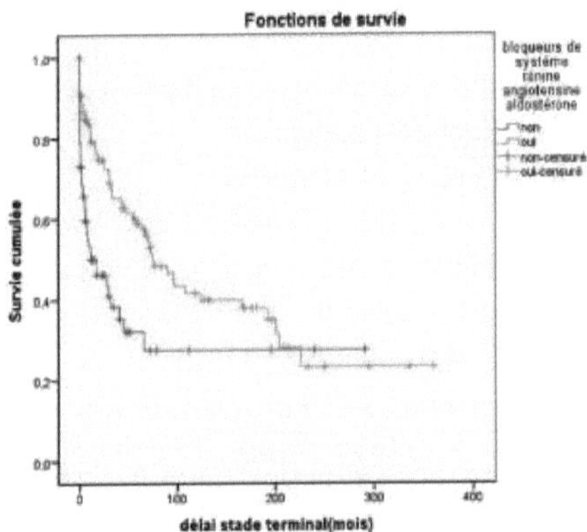

Figure 27: Renal survival as a function of renin angiotensin aldosterone system blocker administration

There was no significant impact of either corticosteroid treatment (whatever the protocol used) or immunosuppressive treatment on renal survival.

3.3.2. Multivariate study:

In order to identify the risk factors independently linked to the event, we conducted a multivariate study using stepwise logistic regression, including the following variables in the first stage: age, sex, smoking, circumstances of discovery of nephropathy, arterial hypertension, initial GFR, 24-hour proteinuria, MEST-C score and use of ARBs and corticosteroids.

This made it possible to identify independent factors in the development of NIgA towards the terminal stage:

- **Advancing age**
- **The discovery of nephropathy following hypertension and/or renal failure**
- **The presence of Tl-2 and 1 histology**

The fortuitous discovery of nephropathy on the basis of urine sediment anomalies was a factor with a good renal prognosis (Table XXIV).

Table XXIII: Renal survival as a function of clinico-biological and histological parameters

	P	*Odds ratio*	*Confidence interval*
Age (Year)	**0,009**	-	-
CDD :			
HTA	**0,049**	2,32	[i,i;5,56]
SU anomalies	**0,024**	**0,318**[a]	[0,11 ;0,88]
IR	**0,041**	3,47	[1,56 ; 12,14]
SI	**0,049**	2,71	[1,09;8,12]
Tl-2	**0,005**	6	[1,71;20,09]

CDD: circumstances of discovery; HTA: arterial hypertension; SU: urinary sediment; IR: renal insufficiency; S: segmental glomerulosclerosis; T: interstitial fibrosis/tubular atrophy;[a] : positive correlation.

4. COMPARATIVE STUDY :

We have carried out a comparative analysis between the two periods of our study:

4.1. First period 1992-2006 including 94 patients

4.2. Second from 2007-2021 including 119 patients.

4.3. Epidemiological factors :

The 1992-2006 period was marked by a clearer male predominance (p=0.03) and by a younger age (p=0.016). On the other hand, the 2007-2021 period was characterised by a higher level of education (p=0.04) (Table XXV).

Table XXIV: Epidemiological characteristics by study period

	1992 - 2006	*2007 - 2021*	*p*
Sex ratio (M/F)	**2,48**	1,38	**0,03***
Level of education: Bac or higher	9,5%	**25,2%**	**0,04***
Professional status: Active	62,7%	61,3%	0,22
Age (Year)	32,1	**36,3**	**0,016***

M: male; F: female

4.4. Clinico-biological characteristics :

During the period 1992-2006, IgA nephropathy was most frequently revealed by macroscopic hematuria (p=0.02). However, in the second period, the most frequent circumstances of discovery were hypertension (p=0.022) and renal failure (p=0.03). During the 2007-2021 period, patients had a higher BMI (p=0.002) and a greater tendency to hyperuricemia (p=0.007).

There was no significant difference when comparing the other clinical and biological parameters (Table XVI).

Table XXV: Clinico-biological characteristics according to study period

	1992 - 2006	*2007 - 2021*	*P*
CDD :			
HU macroscopic	**27,6%**	15,1%	**0,02***
HTA	42,5%	**56%**	**0,022***
SU anomaly	29,8%	26%	0,3
SN	23,4%	21,8%	0,48
Renal insufficiency	60,6%	**74%**	**0,03***
BMI (kg/m)^2	24,2	**26,2**	**0,002***
ffidemes	33%	33,7%	0,56
Uricemia (mmol/1)	384,4	**441,6**	**0,007***

CDD: circumstances of discovery; HU: hematuria; HTA: arterial hypertension; SU: urinary sediment; NS: nephrotic syndrome; BMI: body mass index.

4.5. Histological characteristics :

Segmental glomerulosclerosis (SI) was more prevalent in biopsies taken during the 2007-2021 period (p=0.001).

There was no significant difference when comparing the other histological parameters of the MEST-C score during the two periods (Table XXVII).

Table XXVI: Histological characteristics according to study period.

	1992 - 2006	*2007-2021*	*P*
Ml	57,5%	74%	0,06
El	7,4%	9,2%	0,63
SI	58,5%	**74%**	**0,001***
Tl-2	68%	76,5%	0,2
Cl-2	15%	18,5%	0,48

M: mesangial proliferation; E: endocapillary proliferation; S: segmental glomerulosclerosis; T: interstitial fibrosis/tubular atrophy; C: cellular/fibrocellular crescents.

4.6. Therapeutic and evolutionary parameters:

There was no significant difference in the use of AISIs between the two periods. The use of corticosteroids (p=0.008) and in particular the Pozzi protocol (p<0.001) was greater during the second period.

On the other hand, we did not find any significant difference between the two periods in terms of end-stage CKD, use of ERA and death.

Kidney transplantation was more frequent in the 1992-2006 period (p<0.001).

Table XXVII: Therapeutic and evolutionary characteristics according to study period

	1992-2006	*2007-2021*	*P*
BSRAA	57,3%	56,4%	0,49
Corticotherapy	33%	**50,5%**	**0,008***
Pozzi protocol	6,5%	**58,3%**	**<0,001***
Immunosuppressants	2,1%	3,3%	0,45
IRCT	51%	46,2%	0,28
EER	50%	46,2%	0,38
Kidney transplants	**19,1%**	4,2%	**<0,001***
Deaths	2,12%	0%	0,2

BSRAA: renin angiotensin aldosterone system blockers, CKD: chronic renal failure terminal; EER: extra-renal purification.

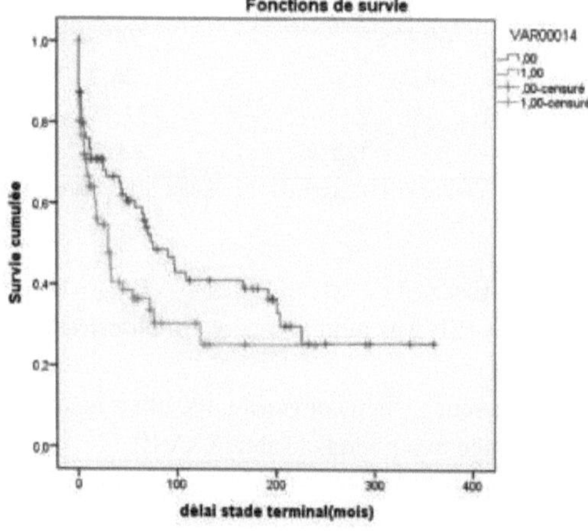

Figure 28: Kidney survival as a function of the period studied

The clinical presentations of NIgA varied from completely asymptomatic forms, revealed by routine urinary examinations (school visits, occupational medicine), to severe forms with rapidly progressive renal failure. Similarly, the histological presentations of NIgA varied, making it difficult to assess and predict the prognosis of this disease.

To this end, we carried out a retrospective descriptive, analytical and comparative study in the internal medicine A department of the Charles Nicolle Hospital in Tunis over a period of thirty consecutive years between 1992 and 2021.

The main aim of our study was to determine the incidence of NIgA over the years in Internal Medicine Department A, and the specific epidemiological, clinico-biological, histological and therapeutic characteristics of this disease. A second important aspect of our study was to analyse patient renal survival as a function of clinical, biological, histological and therapeutic data. This enabled us to understand the influence of these factors on renal prognosis and disease progression in NIgA patients.

Two hundred and thirteen primitive NIgA files were analysed.

The mean age at diagnosis was 34 ±12 years, with extremes ranging from 5 to 80 years. The sex ratio M/F was 1.77.

Familial nephropathy was noted in 39 cases, including 4 cases of IgA nephropathy. Forty-two patients had a history of recurrent ENT infections, and 56 (26%) had unexplored macroscopic haematuria.

The most frequent finding in our population was arterial hypertension (25.4%), followed by macroscopic haematuria (18.8%).

The predominance of hypertension as the circumstance of discovery may be explained by the low GFR in our population. Dietary habits, with a diet rich in sei, and the absence of regular physical activity could also influence this prevalence.

At the time of diagnosis, more than half the patients were hypertensive. Severe grade 3 hypertension was present in more than a third of cases.

On admission, haematuria was macroscopic in 36 patients (17%), microscopic in 137 patients (64.3%) and absent in 40 patients (18.7%).

Biologically, the median 24-hour proteinuria was 2.6g/24h. Nephrotic proteinuria was observed in 46% of the population. Renal failure was present at the time of hospitalisation in 66.7% of patients. The median GFR was 33.9 ml/min/1.73 m^2 SC. Half of our patients had a creatinemia clearance of less than 30 ml/min/1.73 m^2 SC. This severity of renal failure compared with the literature could be explained by the absence of a screening policy and by the indications for PBR. According to the KDIGO recommendations, PBR is performed for proteinuria > 0.5g/24h, whereas in Japan, PBR is performed even for isolated microscopic haematuria.

The lipid profile was disturbed, with hypercholesterolemia in 37.4% of patients and hypertriglyceridemia in 24.8%.

Hyperuricemia was found at the time of diagnosis in 42% of cases. Serum complement assays were performed in 97 patients. We found a fall in the C3 fraction of the complement, a fall in the C1 fraction and a fall in the CH50 in 7%, 2.1% and 13.6% of cases respectively.

Histologically, we found mesangial proliferation (Ml) in 63.8% of biopsies, endo-capillary proliferation (El) in 8.5%, segmental glomerulosclerosis (SI) in 71.4%, interstitial fibrosis/Tl-2 tubular atrophy in 72.8% and Cl and C2 cellular/fibrocellular crescents in 16.9% of biopsies.

Thrombotic microangiopathy was reported in 32% of biopsies. The median Oxford score was 3.

On DFI, diffuse and predominant mesangial lgA binding was noted in all biopsies. Anti-IgM was positive in 63.8% of cases and anti-IgG in 16%. Mesangial C3 complement fixation was observed in 180 patients (84.5%).

Mesangial proliferation (Ml) was correlated with the presence of hypertension ($p=0.008$) and renal failure ($p=0.0045$) at the time the nephropathy was diagnosed.

Endo-capillary proliferation (El) was correlated with age ($p=0.021$), smoking ($p=0.027$), the presence of associated renal failure ($p=0.048$) and hyperuricemia ($p=0.029$).

Segmental glomerulosclerosis (SI) was correlated with high PAS ($p=0.003$) and PAD ($p=0.001$), low glomerular filtration rate ($p<0.001$) and hyperuricemia ($p=0.003$).

Tubular atrophy/interstitial fibrosis (T1-T2) was correlated with male sex ($p=0.04$), smoking ($p=0.007$), presence of hypertension ($p<0.001$), presence of nephrotic syndrome ($p<0.001$) and acute renal failure ($p<0.001$).

The presence of crescents (C1-C2) was correlated with male sex ($p=0.04$) and the presence of renal failure at the time of diagnosis ($p=0.003$).

Fifty-six per cent of patients had гсси renin angiotensin aldosterone system inhibitors. Corticotherapy was prescribed in 91 patients (42.7%), thirty-seven of whom had a Pozzi protocol (40.7%).

Tonsillectomy was performed in 5 cases and no patient had гсси 1 fish oil.

The median follow-up time in our study was 24 months [1-360 months].

Renal survival without progression to CKD was estimated at 83.3% at 1 month, 74.3% at 6 months, 67.2% and 62.9% at 2 years.

The prognostic factors associated with renal survival in univariate analysis were:

- Male gender ($p=0.03$)
- Advancing age ($p=0.049$)
- Smoking ($p=0.012$).
- The presence of hypertension at the time of NIgA diagnosis ($p<0.001$).
- Presence of renal failure at diagnosis ($p<0.001$)
- Proteinuria >2 g/24 ($p<0.001$).
- The presence of hyperuricemia ($p=0.003$).
- The presence at PBR of SI ($p<0.001$), Tl-2 ($p<0.001$), Cl-2 ($p=0.006$) lesions.

In a multivariate study, advanced age, hypertension as the reason for discovery, IR at

the time of diagnosis and the presence of tubular atrophy/interstitial fibrosis and segmental glomerulosclerosis on histology were independent risk factors for recourse to ESRD.
The extra-renal treatment modalities were: hemodialysis (HD) in 83 patients (80.5%) and peritoneal dialysis (PD) in 18 patients (17.4%).
Twenty-three patients underwent renal transplantation. Thirteen patients (56.5%) underwent graft biopsy. PBG was performed in 11 patients for worsening graft function and in 2 patients to investigate isolated proteinuria.
Recurrence of IgA nephropathy was diagnosed in six patients at the end of the course.
We also carried out a comparative analysis between the two periods of our study:

- First period 1992-2006 including 94 patients
- Second period 2007-2021 including 119 patients.
- The 1992-2006 period was marked by a clearer male predominance (p=0.03) and a younger age (p=0.016). The most frequent reason for discovery was macroscopic haematuria (p=0.02). Recourse to renal transplantation was greater during this period (p<0.001).
- In contrast, during the period 2007-2021, IgA nephropathy was more often associated with hypertension (p=0.022) or renal failure (p=0.03). This period was characterised by a higher level of education (p=0.04). Patients had a higher BMI (p=0.002). During this period, hyperuricemia (p=0.007) and segmental glomerulosclerosis (SI) (p=0.001) were more frequent. The prescription of a corticotherapie (p=0,008) and in particular the Pozzi protocol (p<0,001) was more important.

The strength of our work lies in the large number of patients. To our knowledge, this is the first Tunisian study to include 213 patients with IgA nephropathy.
Our study enabled us to :

- Describe the different epidemiological characteristics and clinico-biological presentations of our population.
- Detail the MEST-C score of our patients.
- Assess the renal prognosis, which was fair. In fact, 67% of our patients had IR at the time of diagnosis. This could be explained by recruitment bias.

In the light of our study, we conclude that it is important to encourage mass screening of our population by carrying out a systematic urine test during medical check-ups in the context of school medicine, occupational medicine, recruitment visits and military recruitment visits.
Furthermore, given the impact of genetic and ethnic factors on the severity of renal involvement and progression of IgA nephropathy, we suggest that multicentre Tunisian studies be carried out to better characterise primary IgA nephropathy in our population.

REFERENCES

1. Pillebout E, Verine J. Glomerulonephritis with mesangial immunoglobulin A deposits. Vol. 12, Nephrologie etTherapeutique. Elsevier Masson SAS; 2016. p. 238-54.
2. BergerJ, Hinglais N. Intercapillary deposits of IgA-IgG. J Urol Nephrol (Paris). 1968 Sep;74(9):694-5.
3. HasslerJR. IgA nephropathy: A brief review. Semin Diagn Pathol. 2020 May l;37(3):143-7.
4. Pattrapornpisut P, Avila-Casado *C,* Reich HN. IgA Nephropathy: Core Curriculum 2021. Vol. *78,* American Journal of Kidney Diseases. W.B. Saunders; 2021. p. 429-41.
5. Cattran DC, Coppo R, Cook HT, Feehally J, Roberts ISD, Troyanov S, et al. The Oxford classification of IgA nephropathy: Rationale, clinicopathological correlations, and classification. Kidney Int. 2009 Sep;76(5):534-45.
6. Trimarchi H, BarrattJ, Cattran DC, Cook HT, Coppo R, Haas M, et al. Oxford Classification of IgA nephropathy 2016: an update from the IgA Nephropathy Classification Working Group. Kidney Int. 2017 May l;91(5):1014-21.
7. Ji Y, Yang K, Xiao B, Lin J, Zhao Q, Bhuva MS, et al. Efficacy and safety of angiotensinconverting enzyme inhibitors/angiotensin receptor blocker therapyfor IgA nephropathy: A meta-analysis of randomized controlled trials. J Cell Biochem. 2019 Mar l;120(3):3689-95.
8. Lai KN, Tang SCW, Schena FP, Novak J, Tomino Y, Fogo AB, et al. IgA nephropathy. Nat Rev Dis Primers. 2016 Feb ll;2(16001).
9. Haute Autorite de Sante HAS. Surpoids et obesites de I'adulte : prise en charge medicale de premier recours. Saint-Denis La Plaine; 2011.
10. Abid L, Zakhama L, Trabelsi R, Abdesslem S, Alouane L, Bezdah L, et al. Guide de Pratique Clinique. Prise en charge de I'hypertension arterielle chez I'adulte en Tunisie [Clinical Practice Guidelines. Management of Hypertension in Tunisian Adults], Tunis Med. 2021;99(08- 09):767-847.
11. Bruno Baudin. Nephrotic syndrome. Rev Francoph Lab. 2013 Sep;43(455):51-6.
12. Froissart M, RossertJ, Jacquot *C,* Paillard M, Houillier P. Predictive performance ofthe modification of diet in renal disease and Cockcroft-Gault equations for estimating renal function. Journal of the American Society of Nephrology. 2005;16(3):763-73.
13. Evaluation of glomerular filtration rate and proteinuria for the diagnosis of chronic kidney disease. Nephrology and Therapeutics. 2009;5(4):302-5.
14. Official Journal Ofthe internatiinal Society Of nephrology KDIGO 2012 Clinical Practice Guideline for the Evaluation and Management of Chronic Kidney Disease. Kidney Int Suppl [Internet], 2013;3(l). Available from: www.publicationethics.org
15. HasslerJR. IgA nephropathy: A brief review. Semin Diagn Pathol. 2020 May l;37(3):143-7.
16. Coppo R, Troyanov S, Bellur S, Cattran D, Cook HT, Feehally J, et al. Validation ofthe Oxford classification of IgA nephropathy in cohorts with different presentations and treatments. Kidney Int. 2014Jan l;86(4):828-36.
17. Herzenberg AM, Fogo AB, Reich HN, Troyanov S, Bavbek N, Massat AE, et al. Validation ofthe Oxford classification of IgA nephropathy. Kidney Int. 2011 Aug l;80(3):310-7.
18. Haas M, Verhave JC, Liu ZH, Alpers CE, Barratt J, Becker JU, et al. A multicenter study of the predictive value of crescents in IgA nephropathy. Journal ofthe American Society of Nephrology. 2017;28(2):691-701.
19. Pozzi C, Andrulli S, Del Vecchio L, Melis P, Fogazzi GB, Altieri P, et al. Corticosteroid Effectiveness in IgA Nephropathy: Long-Term Results of a Randomized, Controlled Trial. Journal of the American Society of Nephrology. 2004 Jan;15(l):157-63.
20. Ames J, Onadio VD, Oseph J, Rande PG. IgA NEPHROPATHY. N Engl J Med. 2002 Sep 5;347(10).

Wyld ML, Chadban SJ. Recurrent IgA nephropathy after kidney transplantation. Transplantation. 2016;100(9):1827-32.

APPENDICES

Appendix 1: The different causes of secondary IgA nephropathy (1)

	Causes
Hepatopathy and gastrointestinal diseases	Hepatopathies (alcoholic cirrhosis, chronic viral hepatitis, non-alcoholic hepatic steatosis) emeliac disease, Crohn's disease, hemorrhagic rectocolitis, Whipple's disease
Viral infections	HIV, Cytomegalovirus, Viral hepatitis B, Viral hepatitis C
Other infections	Chronic mucosal infections (streptococcus, staphylococcus), Lyme disease, Chlamydia pneumonia, malaria, schistosomiasis, leprosy, HTLV1
Autoimmune diseases	Ankylosing spondylitis, ANCA vasculitides, rheumatoid arthritis, systemic lupus erythematosus, dermatosis herpetiformis, Sjogren's syndrome, psoriasis, Reiter's syndrome
Respiratory tract	Chronic obstructive pulmonary disease, idiopathic pulmonary fibrosis, bullous lung disease, cystic fibrosis, primary pulmonary hemosiderosis
Neoplasia	IgA myeloma, non-Hodgkin's lymphoma, Hodgkin's lymphoma, cutaneous T-cell lymphoma, lung cancer, renal cell carcinoma

Appendix 2: Data collection form

"Primary IgA nephropathy in adults: epidemiological, clinical, histological and evolutionary profile".

Identification

1) Name /prёпот :
2) Xuinero file:
3) Date of birth :
4) Age on admission :
5) Date of hospitalisation :
6) Sex: male □ /female □
7) Geographical origin : Country/Nationality :
8) Level of education: illiterate □ primary □ secondary □ baccalaureate □ university □ (bac + number of years)
9) Professional status : in training Dactif □ en chomage □ invalided □ retraitd □

MEDICAL HISTORY ;

1) Family antdcddents :
a) Parental consanguinity □
b) Ndphropathy: □
c) Hematuria □
d) HTA □
e) Others :
2) Personal antdcddents :
a) Recurrent ENT infections □
b) Hematuria: microscopic □ macroscopic □/ /recurrent □
c) Diabetes □
d) Hypertension □
e) Heart disease □
f) Allergy □
g) Others :
3) Smoking = yes □ /no □ if yes =Packages/year . smoked since ....
4) Drug addiction: yes □ /no □
5) Alcoholism: yes □ /no □

Circumstances of discovery :

1) Redematous syndrome □
2) HTA □
3) Macroscopic hematuria □

Triggering factor for haematuria :

Interval between the triggering factor and the episode of haematuria:

4) Incidental: urine sediment anomaly □
5) Nephrotic syndrome □
6) Renal insufficiency □

Triggering factors:

1) Infection □
a) Type :

b) Time period preceding the appearance of symptoms of the disease:
2) Taking medication □
a) Therapeutic class :
b) Time before symptoms of the disease appear:
3) Others :

Clinical :

1) Etatgeneral:
2) Weight = kg / height = cm/ BMI=
3) Conjunctive=
4) PAS = PAD =
5) Temperature :
6) Skin signs: □
7) ENT signs □
8) Respiratory signs: □
9) Joint signs: □
10) Digestive signs: □
11) Kidney signs :
a) ffideme : Localise □ Generalise □
b) Hematuria: Microscopic DMacroscopic □
c) Hypertension: Systolic □ Diastolic □
12)Urine strips: Ptu : Hu :

Biology

1) Blood :
   a) Uree :
   b) Creatinine= DFG= ml/min by MDRD
   c) Natremie :
   d) Kaliemie :
   e) Calcemie :
   f) Phosphate :
   g) Bicarbonate :
   h) Protidemie : albuminemia : gamma globulins : al a2 : Pl: P2:
   i) Hemoglobin : VGM : TCMH : GB : platelets :
   j) ALAT: ASAT: GGT: PAL: BT
   k) CRP :
   l) Lipid balance : Cholesterol = Triglycerides =
   m) Uric acid :
   n) Serum IgA :
   o) C3 : C4 : CH50
   p) AAN : anti-DNA :
2) Urine :
   a) Proteinuria: Ptu 24h
   b) Hematuria :
   c) Leukocyturia :

Additional tests :

1) Renal ultrasound :

a) Kidney size: RD =RG=
b) Differentiation :
2) Cardiac ultrasound: LVEF: pericardial effusion □
3) Chest X-ray :

Renal Biopsy Puncture (RBBP)

1) PBR: yes □ no □
2) Date of the PBR: delay in relation to the onset of the disease:
3) Technique: echoguidee □ scannoguidee □
4) Indications for PBR: Isolated Hu □, Isolated IR □, IR with HU without proteinuria □, Ptu24h < 0.5g/24h □, Ptu24h between 0.5 and 3g/24h □, Ptu24h > 3g/24h without SNd, SN □ .
5) Indications for the second PBR :
6) PBR complications: yes □ no □ type: treatment:
7) Glomerular lesions :
a) Total number of glomeruli Number of glomeruli in PAC=
b) Mesangium: mesangial thickening □ Mesangial proliferation □
c) Segmental glomerulosclerosis □ Global glomerulosclerosis □
d) Podocytosis □
e) Endocapillary proliferation □
f) Fibrinoid necrosis □
g) Extra-capillary proliferationD Increasing number of cells= Increasing number of fibrocells= Increasing number of fibrous cells= Increasing number of fibrous cells =
8) Tubulo-interstitial lesions :
a) Interstitial inflammatory infiltrate □
b) Tubular necrosis □
c) Interstitial fibrosis/tubular atrophy □
d) Cylinders □ Type: hyaline □ hematic □ granular □
9) Vascular lesions □
a) Arteriolosclerosis □
b) MAT □
c) Fibrous endarteritis □
10) Oxford classification :
a) Mesangial proliferation: MO □ Ml □
b) Endocapillary proliferation:E0 □ El □
c) Segmental glomerulosclerosis :S0 □ SI □
d) Tubular atrophy / interstitial fibrosis: TO ΠT1 ΠT2 □
e) Cell/fibro-cell crescents:C0 □ Cl □ C2 □
11) Immunofluorescence :
a) Lg A mesangial deposits □
b) IgM deposits □
c) IgG deposits □
d) C3 depots □
e) DepotdeClqD
f) Depot de chaines legeres □ type : lambda □ kappa □

Treatment:

1) Conservative treatment :
a) Smoking cessation □
b) Fluid restriction □
c) Lipid-lowering treatment □ type:

d) Treatment of hyperuricemia □
e) Nephroprotective treatment □ ACE inhibitors □ ARAIIs □
2) Antihypertensive treatment (therapeutic class):
a) IEC □type :
b) ARAII □ type:
c) icm
d) Diuretics □
e) Central antihypertensive □
f) Alpha bioquant □
g) Beta bioquant □
3) Antibiotic treatment :
a) Therapeutic class :
b) Indication:
c) Time to infection
4) Tonsillectomy □
5) Fish oil □
6) Corticosteroid treatment : Date treatment started:
a) Indication:
b) Protocol: oral corticosteroid therapy □ Pozzi protocol □
7) Cyclophosphamide :
a) Circumstance of addition: Firstly □ Secondly □
b) Dose :
c) Indication:
8) Other treatments presented :
9) Treatment complications:
a) Metabolic :
b) Infectious diseases :
c) Tumoral :

Evolution :

Evolution	1 month	3 months	6 months	1 YEAR	18 months	2 years	End of monitoring
Uree							
Creatininemia							
Protidemie							
24-hour proteinuria							
Hematuria							
HTA							

1) Follow-up period :
2) Therapeutic compliance: yes □ no □
3) Kidney function :
a) Clearance :
b) Stage 1 renal failure :
4) End stage :
a) Not achieved □
b) D'emblde □
c) Progression □ ddlai :
5) Extra-renal purification :
a) Hemodialysis: □

b) Peritoneal dialysis : □
c) Date of first performance :
6) Lost track of: yes □ no □
7) Deeds :
d) Cause of ddees :
e) Deadline :
8) Kidney transplants :
a) Preemptive: □ At stage5 of CKD □ Not done □
b) Anёe:
c) donor: living □ /cadavdric □
d) HLA typing: donor: recipient :
e) Delay from start of EER :
f) Induction treatment :
g) Maintenance treatment:
h) Duration of follow-up :
i) Evolution : Proteinuria : hematuria : renal function :
j) PBG: yes □ no □ Date: indications :
k) NIgA relapse yes □ no □ time to onset compared to RT :

Appendix 3: Activation pathways of the complement system(142)

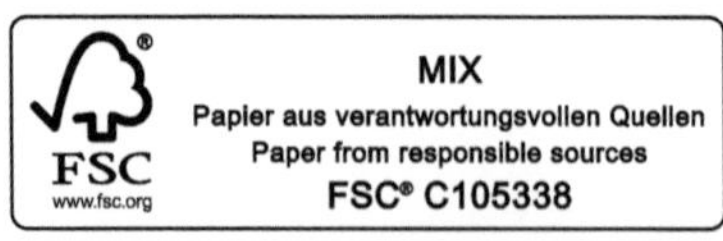

Printed by Books on Demand GmbH, Norderstedt / Germany